THE ROLE OF
AUTONOMICS
IN THE ORIGIN AND HEALING OF
CHRONIC ILLNESS

PRAISE FOR
THE NEUROBIOLOGY OF CONNECTION

Truly a masterwork, this is a rare combination of scientific insight, spiritual wisdom, and practical tools for daily life. Beautifully written, it's warm and inviting, like a clear path through green forest groves. Poetic, personal, comprehensive, and endlessly useful, in these pages you're in the company of a brilliant and warm-hearted guide to lasting well-being, love, and inner peace.

-RICK HANSON, PH.D.,
AUTHOR OF BUDDHA'S BRAIN: THE PRACTICAL NEUROSCIENCE OF HAPPINESS, LOVE, AND WISDOM

"A marvelous text, full of brilliant transdisciplinary insights!"

-DARCIA NARVAEZ, PHD
PROFESSOR EMERITA OF PSYCHOLOGY, DEVELOPER OF THE EVOLVED NEST

"A perfect bridge between neuroscience and the wisdom traditions."

-JD DANIELS, MD, MPH
PROFESSOR OF FAMILY & COMMUNITY MEDICINE, ASST DEAN OF STUDENTS FOR SIU MEDICINE

"The origin story of human connectedness is not frozen in deep time. It is here, alive, in our present-now, with pulse and with resonance so deep that in somehow coming into contact with this book, I am simultaneously coming more into contact with this pulse. Gabriel's ability to dissolve limiting paradigms allows the reader to dissolve them, too - reconfiguring our own origin story. This is a book for any human interested in vitality, interested in decoding wellbeing, and interested in coming home."

-JORDHYNN GUY, CCC
DEVELOPER OF THE ELITE RESILIENCE FRAMEWORK

"Gabriel has brought together some of the cutting-edge work in autonomic physiology, neurobiology and neuroscience within the broader context of late-stage capitalism. Healing in absence of context can amplify trauma. This book attempts to address the decontextualization of modern science, and in the process, engages the reader in deep neural cartography for troubled times. This work is pioneering the emerging field of what Gabriel calls connection phenomenology. It is timely and necessary."

—ALNOOR LADHA
CO-AUTHOR OF POST CAPITALIST PHILANTHROPY: HEALING WEALTH IN THE TIME OF COLLAPSE

"Neurobiology of Connection is a book we all need—a user's manual for our nervous systems. Brilliantly insightful and practical, we can learn to understand why we are the way we are moment-to-moment, meet our needs in ways that heal old traumas, and enhance deep connection with other humans and the world around us. Gabriel brings together material from indigenous cultures, neuroscience, neurochemistry, mindfulness, somatically-informed trauma work, Polyvagal Theory, and literature, combined with attention to his inner world, in order to create an updated model of the Autonomic Nervous System. I have made so many changes to the way I teach, and my students are loving it!"

—MARCIA MILLER
CERTIFIED YOGA THERAPIST, REIKI MASTER TEACHER, SENIOR TEACHER FOR UZIT

"My first nervous system health mentor introduced me to both Polyvagal Theory and the concept of 'cellular safely'. As a bodyworker practicing Visceral Manipulation through a trauma and nervous system lens, I use the sensitivity of my hands to introduce cellular safety to decontextualized stress responses (also known as tension) in the body. From the release of tension anchored in safety, systemic well-being emerges and continues to emerge as the body continues to be approached and supported in this way. It has been a challenge to find my work accurately represented through a lens of neurobiology. I am beyond grateful for this eloquent expansion of Polyvagal Theory that brings in the knowing of my hands and the wisdom that flows from our bodies to our heart, then our brain.

I also deeply appreciate Gabriel for naming the domination mindset that is imbedded into the fabric of modernity and for challenging the status quo around it. It is bold and necessary."

-KELLEY CURTIS
BODYWORKER AND NERVOUS SYSTEM HEALTH PRACTITIONER

"Gabriel has waved a poetic wand over off-putting medical-speak and pulled the curtain back on the divine delighting herself in her magic shop. In this monumental work that is being constructed through him, I get to press my nose against that glass. I tell people the work Gabriel is conducting is the science behind safety. Bravo maestro! A Slam Dunk."

-JIMBO GRAVES,
AUTHOR OF TILLAGE

The Neurobiology of Connection is a breathing, moving testimony to the profound magic our bodies, with our autonomic nervous systems as creative center, eternally weave. This book pierces the layers of patriarchy and disembodied control that dominate much of the current scientific discourse. Gabriel's brilliant writing and insights are equally grounded in neuroscience and deep timeless inquiry, and offer the essential map to the dance of wholeness and connection we all own as birthright.

-DR. AMBER ELIZABETH L GRAY,
HUMAN RIGHTS PSYCHOTHERAPIST, SOMATIC & DANCE/MOVEMENT THERAPIST, AUTHOR, EDUCATOR, & WILD WARRIOR

"Gabriel's work with the autonomic nervous system offers powerful keys to understanding how to participate in relational spaces that consciously nurture trusting relationships and invite creativity. These are key ingredients for the kind of ongoing attunement we need to generate a culture of care, belonging, and collective wellbeing. The neurobiology of connection is a wide open gateway to inform the awareness of human connection that is essential to create contexts for diverse people to come together and navigate the many complex, intersecting challenges we face as a species on this planet. If you recognize the importance of lived experience on our ability to form healthy relationships with ourselves and others, build community and collaborate for social and environmental change, this body of work offers an embodied, highly functional map to actively heal the fractured social territory of our times."

-CARRI MUNN
FOUNDING PARTNER, CIRCLE GENERATION

BY NATUREZA GABRIEL

The Neurobiology of Connection

Hearth Science

Autonomic Compass

Autonomic Triage

Restorative Practices of Wellbeing

Keywords: A Field Guide to the Missing Words

So, About that Death Cult you Joined?

The Archeology of Shadows

Sport of Kings

Can't Get Home (Stories)

Destoryer of Empire (Collected Poems 2020-2022)

Origin Stories for Children

THE ROLE OF
AUTONOMICS
IN THE ORIGIN AND HEALING OF
CHRONIC ILLNESS

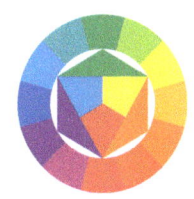

NATUREZA GABRIEL

AUTHOR OF THE NEUROBIOLOGY OF CONNECTION

THE ROLE OF AUTONOMICS IN THE ORIGIN AND HEALING OF CHRONIC ILLNESS
NATUREZA GABRIEL

© 2025 Jaguar Imprints of Hearth Science, Inc. & Gabriel Kram

All rights reserved. No part of this book may be reproduced or transmitted in any form or by any means, electronic or mechanical, including photocopying and recording, or in any information storage or retrieval system without the prior written permission of Hearth Science. Many of the images in this book are licensed from Unsplash.com

Published by:
Jaguar Imprints
PO Box 567, Nicasio, CA 94946, USA

A CIP record for this book is available from the Library of Congress Cataloging-in-Publication Data

A NOTE FOR READERS

This handbook is part of a series on the application of Autonomics to our lives.

The first handbook in the series, *Autonomic Compass*, lays the general groundwork for understanding core concepts of Autonomics, including what the Autonomic Nervous System is, neuroception, what autonomic states are, and the basic neurology and neurochemistry of autonomic systems. In this volume, we look specifically at the application of the framework to chronic illness.

Because I don't wish to re-write foundation material that I have covered in-depth elsewhere, I direct you to that other volume for a general overview.

If you would like to read the core pedagogy of Autonomics, rather than or in addition to focusing on its application, I direct you to the Autonomics Trilogy: *The Neurobiology of Connection*, *Ground*, and *Body as Verb*.

Warmly,
Gabriel

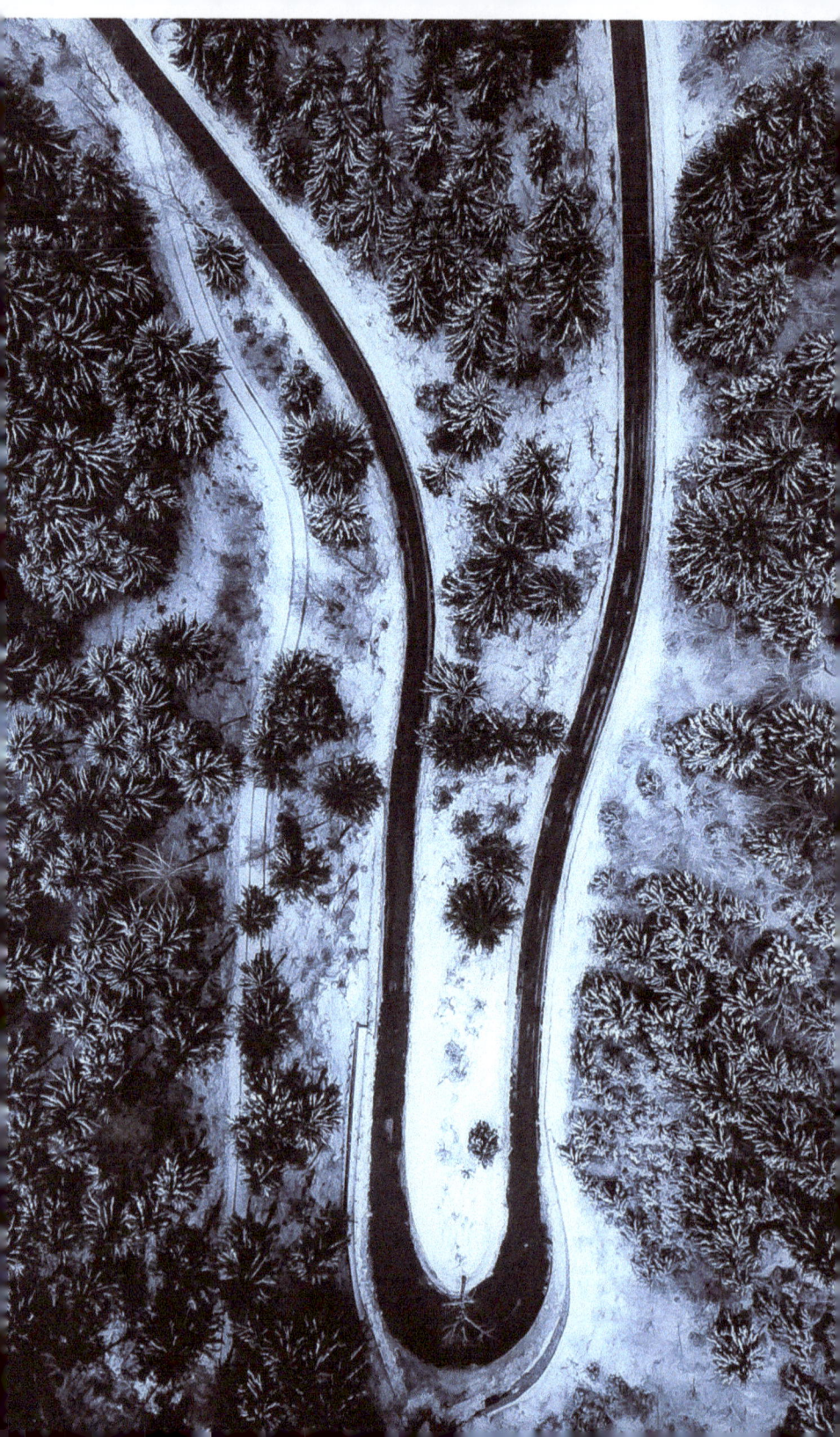

TABLE OF CONTENTS

Glossary — 16
Illustrations — 18
Autonomic Mandala — 20
Introduction — 22

PART ONE: FOUNDATIONS

01- San Rafael — 29
02- Take Two — 33
03- Early Experiences — 37
04- Bumper Stickers — 39
05- Sound Engineer — 42
06- Synthesis — 47
07- ACES — 49
08- The Fight-Flight Responses — 54
09- Digestive Difficulties & Lifethreat Responses — 63
10- The Difference between Freeze & Shutdown — 69
11- Three Variants of Lifethreat Response — 71

PART TWO: FRAMEWORKS

12- Self as Water — 77
13- Mindbody System — 80
14- It's Not in Your Head — 83
15- Ecological Model — 85
16- Relating — 89
17- Autonomic Self — 91

18- Body as Compass   95

PART THREE: APPLICATION

19- Practicing Something New   97
20- Metabolizing Allostatic Loads   100
21- Getting Alternative Stress Responses on the Menu   105
22- Boundary Setting & Chronic Illness   112
23- Not Eating Other People's Waste Energy   117
24- Placate   122
25- Getting Other Defensive Responses Back   127
26- Evoking Connection States   134
27- Conclusion   137

APPENDIX ONE: SOMATICALLY-ORIENTED TRAUMA HEALING LINEAGES AND INTERVENTIONS WITH OVERLAP TO AUTONOMICS   140

APPENDIX TWO: PRACTICES FOR EVOKING CONNECTION STATES IN NO PARTICULAR ORDER   144

GLOSSARY

Appease: a defensive autonomic state characterized by responding to a threat using elements of social neurology (Connection System) and social neurochemistry.

Autonomic State: An energy-processing template of the Autonomic Nervous System (ANS) that governs how experience flows through and across our bodymind.

Connection System: One of the three foundational autonomic neurological systems, the Connection System is the most recently evolved of our core autonomic systems. In the presence of a felt sense of safety, the Connection System unites the neural regulation of the face, voice, eyes, the tuning of the middle ear, and the hands with the heart and breath, allowing us to come into attuned connection with another. The Connection System undergirds salugenic (health-creating) autonomic states. For students of Polyvagal Theory, this is known as the Social Engagement or Ventral Vagal System.

Grounding System: One of the three foundational autonomic neurological systems, the Grounding System is the most ancient of our core autonomic systems. This system is organized through the unmyelinated sub-diagrphagmatic Vagus, and located primarily between the bottom of the rib cage and the pelvic floor. This system, under the chemistries of life-threat (endogenous opioids) undergirds autonomic shutdown responses, which are always implicated in chronic illness, via interface with the immune and endocrine systems. For students of Polyvagal Theory, this is known as the Dorsal Vagal System, although Polyvagal Theory fails to understand the role of this system in health-creation.

Interoception: The Mother of all senses, interoception is our ability to feel ourselves from inside. I'm calling it the Mother of All Senses, because the Autonomic Nervous System can co-operate with, or co-opt all of your extero-senses (vision, hearing, smell, taste, touch) and put them in service to the ANS.

Neuroception: the moment-to-moment neural detection of safety, danger, or lifethreat by the embodied nervous system

Movement System: One of the three foundational autonomic neurological systems, the Movement System evolved with the vertebrate body plan. It places the autonomous motor control of appendages close to the specific limb, in Central Pattern Generators (CPGs) located in a series of post-synaptic ganglia running up and down the spine. It also includes brainstem CPGs that regulate sucking, swallowing, and breathing, as well as components of the vestibular and ocular systems required to sense the location of the body in space. This system, under the chemistries of danger (adrenaline and cortisol) undergirds autonomic fight-or-flight responses, and is called the Sympathetic Nervous System in orthodox neurology, although this naming fails to recognize the role of the system in health-creating states.

Placate: A defensive autonomic state characterized by responding to a lifethreat using elements of social neurology (Connection System) and social neurochemistry. A core autonomic pattern in chronic illness.

SIMPLIFIED ILLUSTRATION OF THE THREE PRIMARY AUTONOMIC SYSTEMS

CONNECTION SYSTEM IN BLUE

MOVEMENT SYSTEM IN YELLOW

GROUNDING SYSTEM IN RED

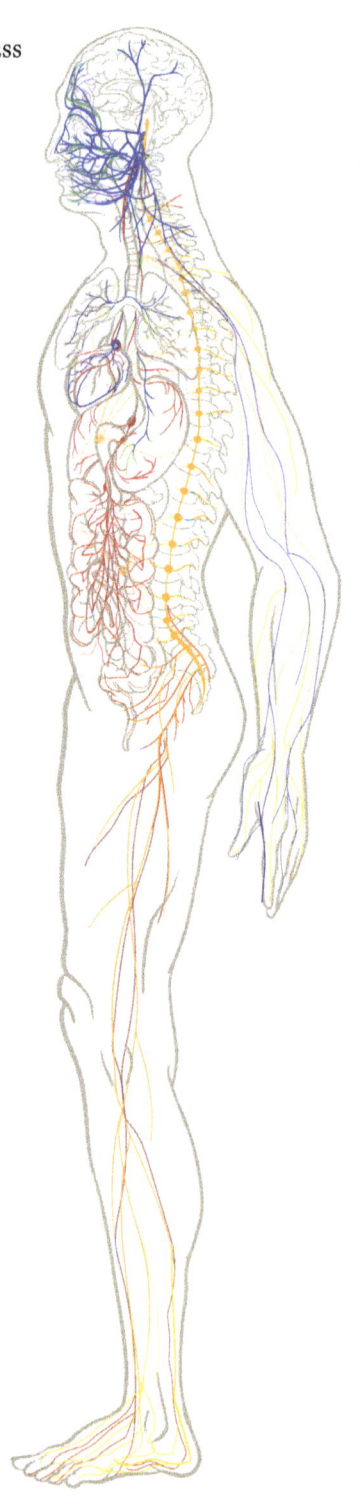

ILLUSTRATION OF THE THREE PRIMARY NEUROCEPTIONS OF SAFETY, DANGER, AND LIFETHREAT, WITH THEIR CORRELATION TO STATES OF LIQUID WATER, STEAM, AND ICE.

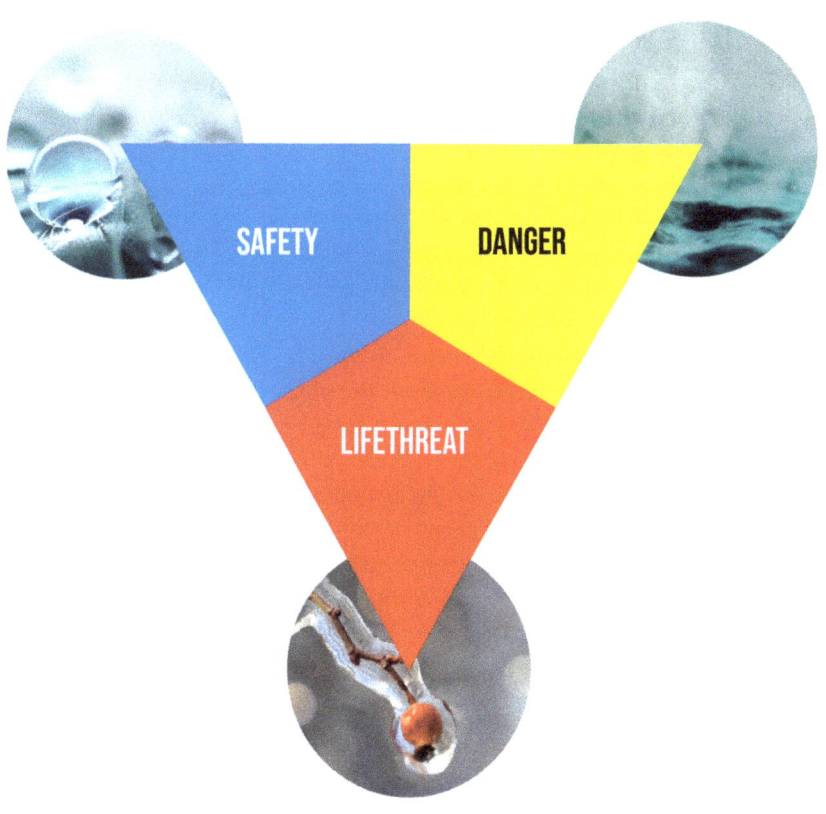

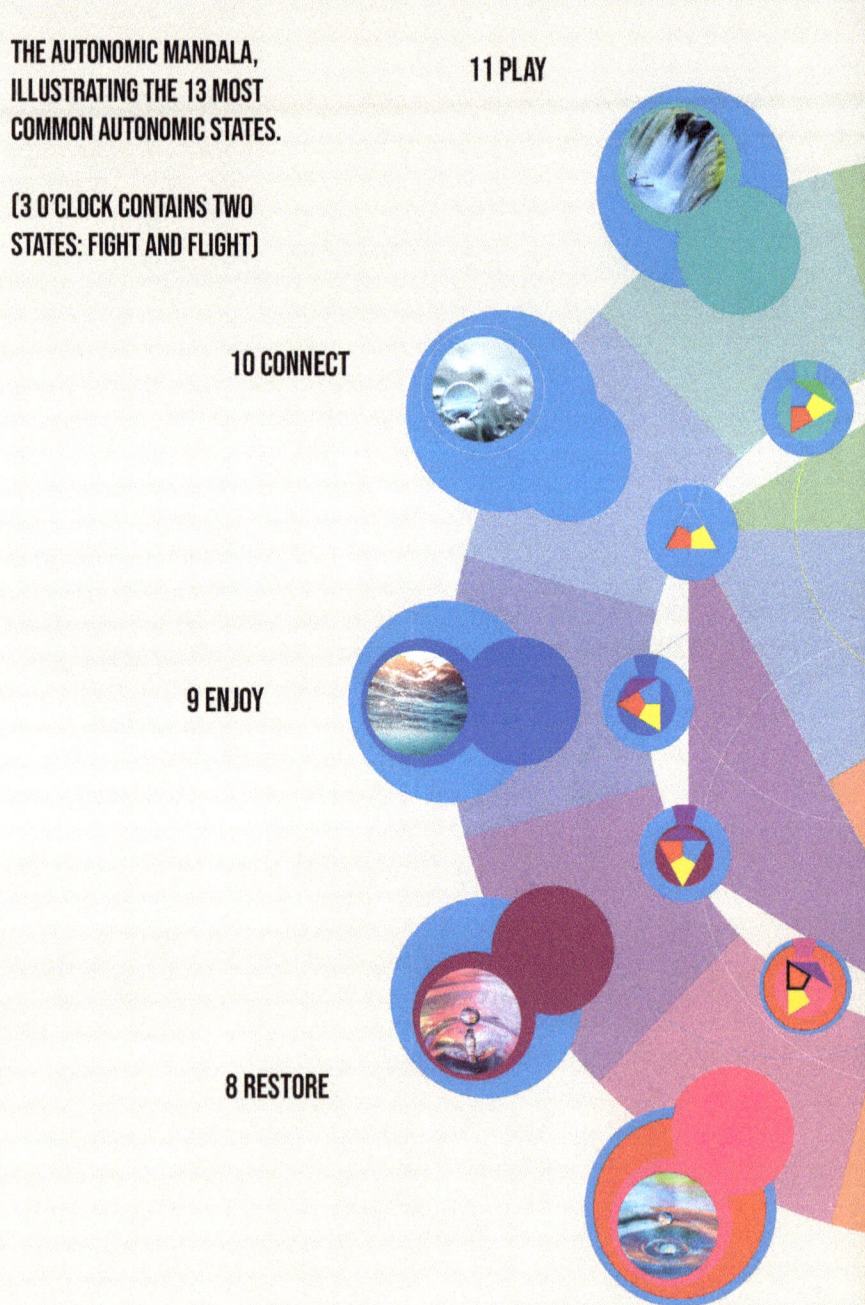

THE AUTONOMIC MANDALA, ILLUSTRATING THE 13 MOST COMMON AUTONOMIC STATES.

(3 O'CLOCK CONTAINS TWO STATES: FIGHT AND FLIGHT)

1 ACCOMMODATE

2 APPEASE

3 FIGHT / FLIGHT

4 FREEZE

5 PLACATE

6 SHUTDOWN

HEALTH CREATING STATES FROM 8 TO 12 O'CLOCK. DANGER STATES FROM 2 TO 3 O'CLOCK, LIFETHREAT STATES FROM 4 TO 6 O'CLOCK. 1 AND 7 O'CLOCK CAN BE HEALTH CREATING OR DISEASE CREATING DEPENDING ON CONTEXT

INTRODUCTION

The diagnosis and treatment of complex chronic illness is an art as much as it is a science. Chronic illness develops as the complex non-linear interaction of numerous physiological systems, including the neurological, immune, and endocrine.

It is often pre-conditioned by early life and adverse childhood experiences, yet can ultimately emerge in response to either endogenous or exogenous factors.

People can develop chronic illness as a result of exposure to environmental chemistry (toxicity), mold, or tick-borne illness. It can develop as the result of a virus (e.g. COVID-19) or other kind of infection. It can develop in the wake of a life change that is unduly stressful, a breakup, or the loss of a loved one. Two people may have identical exposures, living for example in a house with a mold problem, and one person may develop chronic illness while the other is unaffected.

This book is therefore but a piece in a larger puzzle. No one with chronic illness develops it without their Autonomic Nervous System (ANS) playing a causal role. It is not always *THE* primary cause, but it is always implicated in some way, because the Autonomic Nervous System governs the energy processing templates through which our experience flows, and *complex chronic illness is both a cause and a result of sustained experiences of lifethreat*.

If you have some form of complex chronic illness, and you are reading this book, you are likely aware of the degree to which mainstream allopathic medicine will have difficulty making sense of your experience. Allopathic medicine's conceptualization of disease is quite mechanistic. It still views the various organ systems in the body as being akin to the parts of a car. It then has specialists (cardiologists, neurologists, gastro-enterologists) that work on these various parts. This divide-and-conquer approach, which is of imperial origin, is ill-suited to any stress-related disorder or injury, for the simple reason that the systems that mediate the stress response are mind-body systems. The Autonomic Nervous System, which is the neural architecture of the mind-body connection, governs the organ function of *all physiological systems* based on our moment-to-moment detection of safety, danger, or lifethreat.

You can have a problem in your guts, and the gastro-enterologist can be looking very intently at this organ and diagnosing its dysfunction, as manifest through digestive difficulties, disrupted peristaltic rhythm, altered gut PH, and changes to the microbiome. But what your gastro-enterologist does not understand, and is not looking at, is that often the issues in the gut did not originate in the gut, but in the *neural regulation* of the gut. In plain language, your Autonomic Nervous System turned off your guts. And this means that the switch for turning them back on is not in your guts, even if your primary symptoms reside there.

Chronic illness, furthermore, is not simply a feature of the Autonomic Nervous System, but rather develops in the interactions between your immune system, nervous system, and endocrine system. Modern medicine and science understand very little about the immune system.

Bob Naviaux MD PhD, a pioneer in mitochondrial medicine who runs the Naviaux Lab at the University of California San Diego, recently conducted a set of tests on adults with myalgic encephalomyelitis/chronic fatigue syndrome (ME/CFS) and measured the presence of 500 molecules in their blood.[1] While 25% of the molecular signatures of the disease overlap between people who have it, 75% of the molecular signatures do not. This is to say that even among people who have the same chronic illness, in this case ME/CFS, the actual metabolomics of the disease are quite individual and varied.

---

1 https://naviauxlab.ucsd.edu/science-item/chronic-fatigue-syndrome-research/

If you have chronic illness, you don't really have a *category* of illness. You have your own unique illness with its own unique molecular expresssion. Every chronic illness is an N of 1. While this is profoundly, and sometimes endlessly frustrating, it means that in order to heal you must be actively engaged in the detective work of unraveling the illness. As the person living in the body with the illness, you are the most expertly positioned to engage in sense-making around it. You know how it feels to be in your body. You are aware of when you feel better, and when you feel worse, and the particular patterns of symptoms. No one else in the world, no matter howsoever expert they might be, approaches your level of direct experience of what is happening.

In order to participate actively in your own healing, it is useful to understand the various physiological systems involved, and what I'll try to do in this handbook is give you a sense of how the Autonomic Nervous System functions (or rather how its functioning degrades) in chronic illness, and some of the fundamental patterns we have noticed in working with patients and clients with chronic illness, as well as assisting and consulting with other practitioners serving these populations. What I am going to focus on here, ultimately, is the degree to which chronic illness is a manifestation of specific defensive patterns of relating. When we develop chronic illness, we get very focused on what is happening *inside* the body. Yet the genesis of chronic illness is almost always traceable to what happens *between* bodies, in the autonomic habits of our relating to others. This is an important reframe in understanding where and how we can intervene with ourselves to move back in the direction of wellbeing. *The symptoms of chronic illness are inside us, but the levers that drive it are between us.*

As you work in the direction of healing, something else to bear in mind is that while it is likely important to address a number of different aspects of the illness in the movement towards healing, the order in which you address different components matters. At some point along your healing pathway you will likely be dealing with infections/ co-infections, inflammatory responses, the gut microbiome, the Autonomic Nervous System, and how your attention works. Each of these are facets of the total experience. Yet you have to find a sequence of addressing these facets that your body responds to. Attention training doesn't work effectively if you have brain fog, or if the distress signals from the body are too strong. It is very difficult, and probably not useful, to try to learn to meditate if you are experiencing acute anxiety.

So as you work with the different facets of your healing process, if something is not yeilding results, move on to something else. It may not be that the area you are working on is not relevant: it may simply be that the timing is not right. This logic clearly holds for this book. For some of you reading it, this will be a timely piece, the next piece, of the puzzle. For some of you reading this, the information it contains will be helpful at some point in the future. If it doesn't resonate, just set it down. It may at some point in the future.

Finally, I would like to confess that I'm not really qualified to write this. I'm not saying that to be humble, but rather because it is true. While I am profoundly expert in the Autonomic Nervous System, I am not profoundly expert in the treatment of chronic illness. I happen to have had the experience of sucessfully transforming chronic illness in myself many years ago, so I can stand on the ground of this lived experience. And I happen to be in regular conversation with several brilliant colleagues who are deeply expert in the treatment of complex chronic illness.

This book arose out of a call-and-response dialogue with one of them. I would not have taken the time to write it if I didn't think it would be at least a little bit useful to some people. That said, this volume is provisional at best: a mere sketch. I confess that part of my hope in getting these notes down is that this will spur my colleague to writing a much more comprehensive treatment of the topic himself.

I know from experience that one of the most psychologically challenging aspects of chronic illness is the slow pace of healing. I think it is important to remember that these illness typically develop over decades. They often trace back to our earliest childhood patterns of relating to caregivers. So while the onset of symptoms can feel sudden and suprising, their genesis is actually of an extremely long duration. I find this important in calibrating our expectations about healing. Part of the challenge in learning to heal is to help your bodymind re-write the scripts of how it responds to threatening experience. And this transformation does not happen in our thinking, but rather deeper down in the body, and deeper down in the nervous system. You are learning to retrain the deeper animal, and in order to do this you have to learn to communicate with these deeper parts of self in the language that they speak.

In our work at Hearth Science we call this developing *autonomic fluency*. It is, truthfully, learning a new language of the felt. This language is also, paradoxically, very ancient. This language is inward (interoceptive to be precise), and it is infinitely nuanced: the primal meaning-making language of the body. To become aware of it will put you into contact with the very depths of Self. Healing is, therefore, a journey of self-discovery, and a journey of transformation.

I therefore wish you patience, and I wish you flourishing vitality. May you feel the deepest sense of safety; may you find and unlock the doors that open upon your own deep wellsprings of wellbeing.

Natureza Gabriel
Founder, Hearth Science
25 April 2025

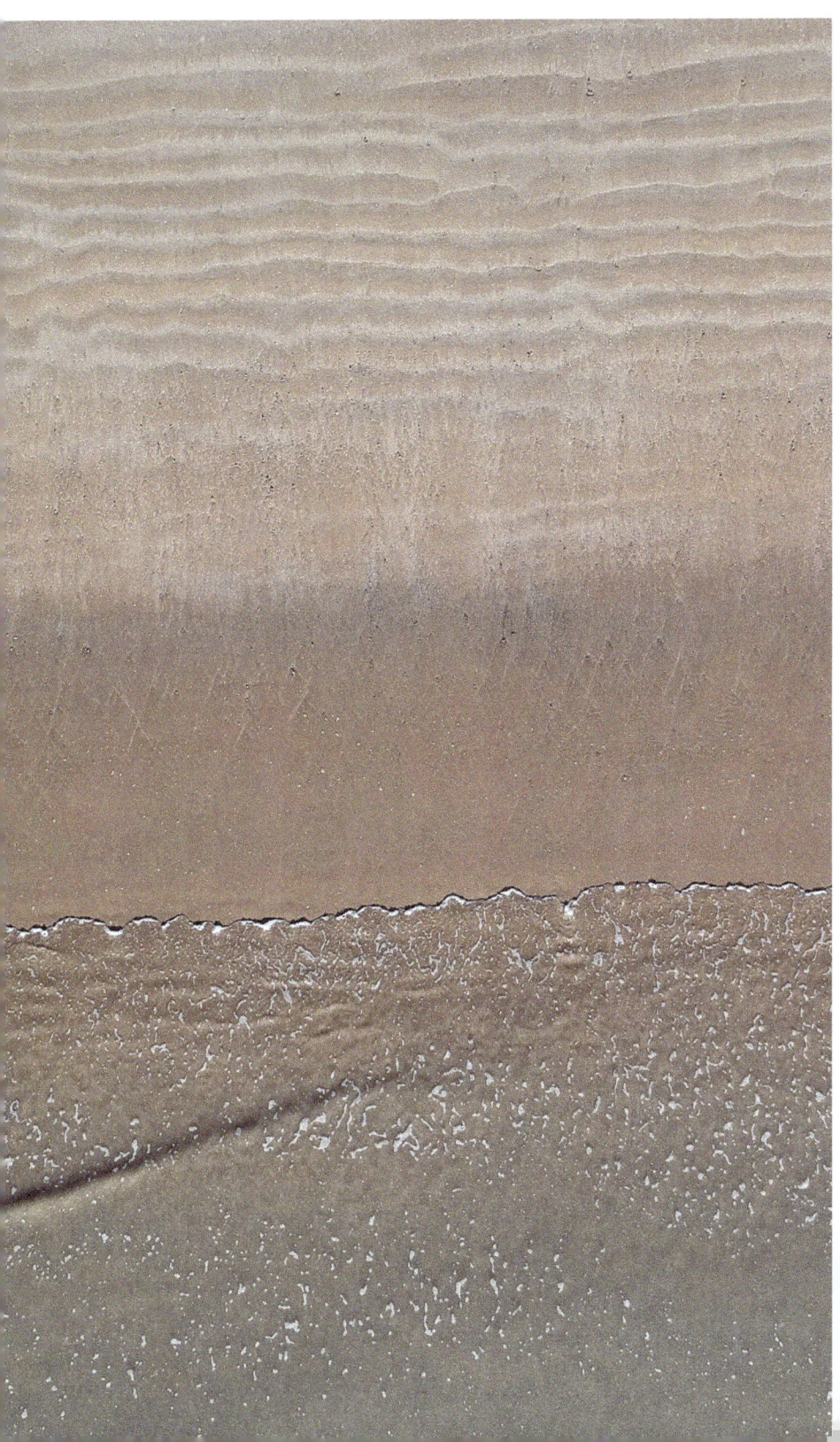

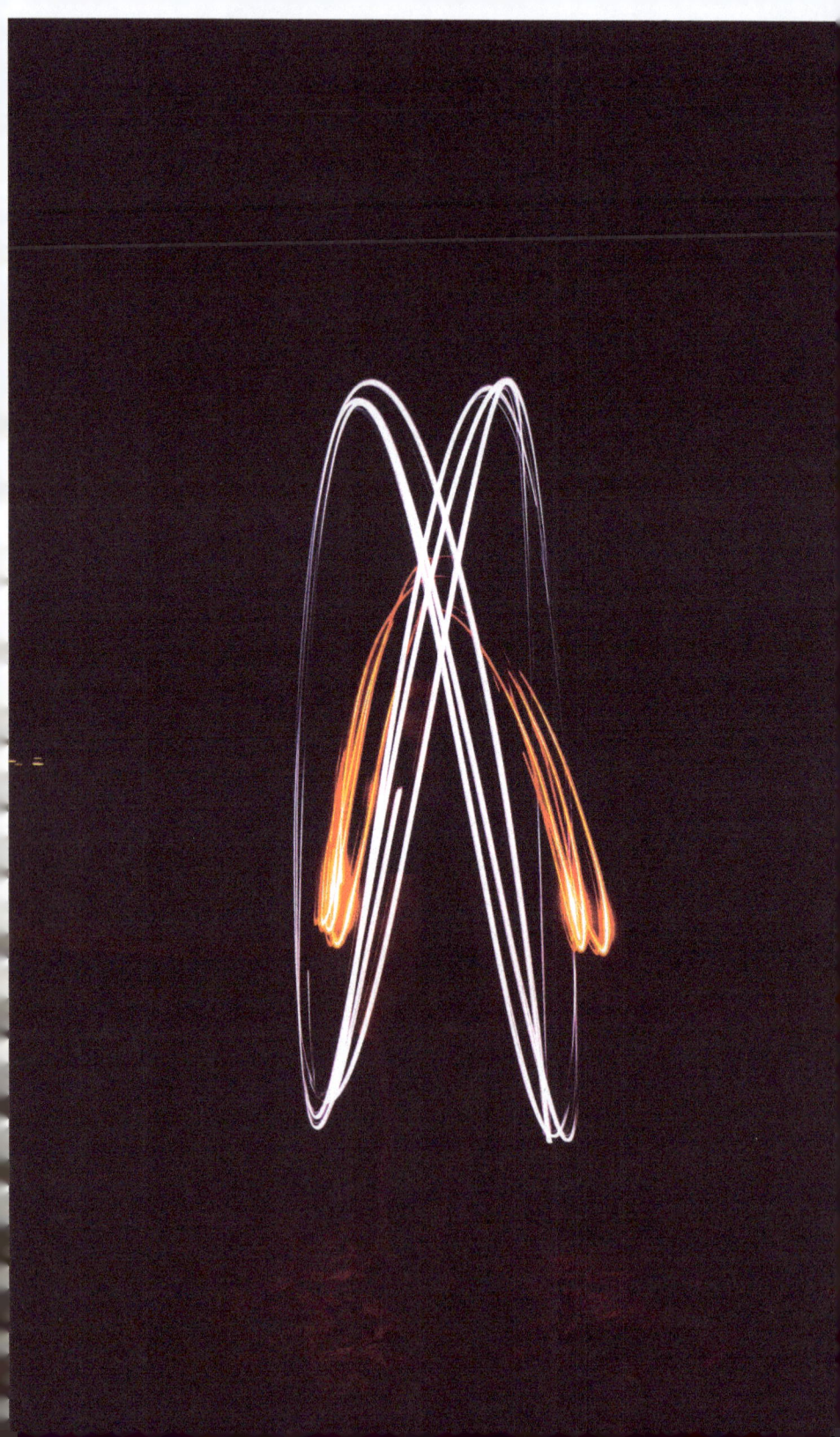

PART ONE: FOUNDATIONS

01- SAN RAFAEL

In the spring of 2024, Bob Naviaux, who runs the mitochondrial cell laboratory at the University of California San Diego introduced me to Dr. Eric Gordon, a functional medicine doctor who specializes in treating complex chronic illness. Bob, who is one of the world's leading practitioners of mitochondrial medicine made this introduction after a long conversation we had about the role of autonomic physiology in the origin and progression of chronic illness. Over the last several years, he had been writing about a phenomenon called the Cell Danger Response, a kind of localized cellular response in the body that in many ways mimics autonomic danger responses that happen systemically. In this response, cells at the site of an injury or wound begin dumping Adenosine Triphosphate (ATP) which is ordinarily used as their primary fuel, into the extra-cellular matrix, where it becomes toxic.

Mitochondria are our cellular engines. Once upon a time, these tiny organelles were other organisms entirely: several billion years ago early single-celled eukaryotic creatures developed a symbiotic relationship with them that has led to one of the most enduring marriages fundamental to the flourishing of life. The cells provided an ideal home for the mitochondria; in exchange the mitochondria power our cells. These tiny engines run on ATP, which is a primary energy currency for metabolic processes, powering the contraction of muscles, the propagation of nerve impulses, and various kinds of chemical synthesis.

The Cell Danger Response that Bob has noted and studied is

perplexing, because when it happens cells take this precious fuel and start dumping it overboard. Intriguingly, outside of the context of the cell, this fuel is toxic, and one of the strange effects of this now extra-cellular ATP (e-ATP) is that it creates a sort of local rogue island around the site of injury that becomes unresponsive to signals of safety from the Central Nervous System: a very unusual effect.

When he told me this story for the first time, I imagined a motorboat and cans of gasoline. I know this is probably not a perfect analogy, but I remember filling boat motors as a kid, and that if you were not careful, sometimes an irridescent sheen of gas would dribble out of the motor and end up on the water. I always felt slightly sick when this happened. Inside the motor, the fuel would power the engine. Outside of the motor, this prismatic sheen of fuel would poison the water. When Bob explained the response to me, this is what I thought of. We are mostly water; more than 70%. Our body is in many ways an inward ocean, and I could see how this response would diffuse into a local area in the body, spreading away from the injured site.

I have spent the past 30 years studying the human nervous system, and the past fifteen focused exclusively on developing a new living model of autonomic physiology called Autonomics. As Bob described the Cell Danger Response, I felt the hair on my arms begin to stand up. It was as though he was describing a tiny fractal of processes of autonomic physiology I had been studying, writing about, and working with clinically for years. A fractal is a mathematical figure that is similar at varying levels of scale. Even if you've never heard this word, you know what a fractal is. Have you ever looked closely at the pattern of run-off from a puddle? And then have you ever been in an airplane and looked down at a river delta from altitude? They create the same patterns. Nature speaks in a pattern language, and the patterns hold true at different scales, from the minute to the immense. The branching of certain trees has the same structure as the branching of the vascular system in your body;

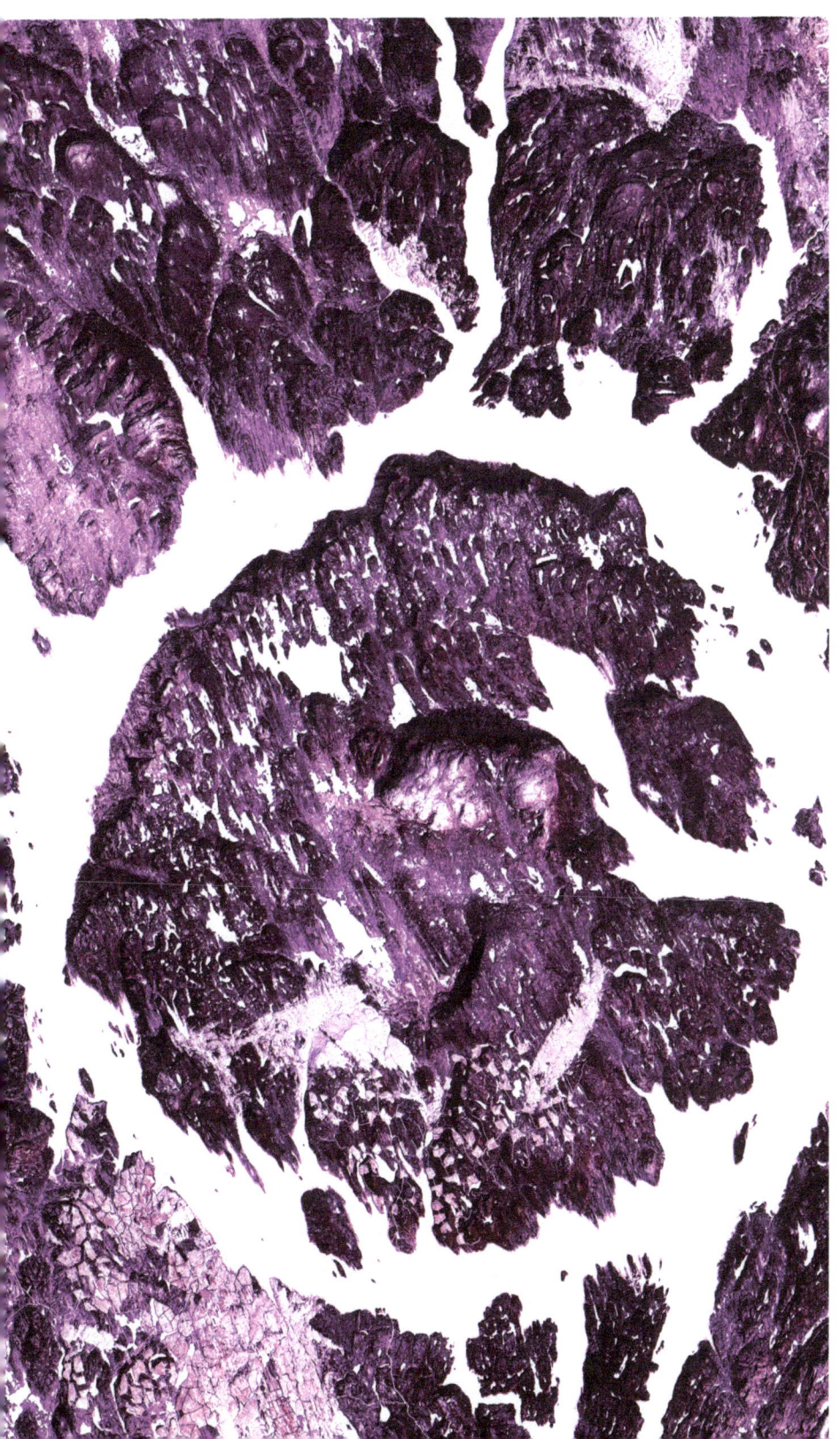

the spiral of a chambered nautilus maps to the geometry of a sunflower which can also be found in the shape of the swirling arm of a galaxy. As Bob described the response I found myself once again in awe of the majesty and mystery of the human body as an expression of the design language of Nature.

The Autonomic Nervous System in the body works in ways similar to the Cell Danger Response. When we are in a salugenic, or health-creating state, the Autonomic Nervous System orchestrates a profound harmonization of our three primary autonomic systems coordinated around the rhythmic pulse of safety, producing the deep neural foundations of wellbeing. But if the Autonomic Nervous System gets shifted into enduring danger or lifethreat responses, and is unable to shift out of them, there are clear and repeatable neurobiological sequelae of this shift that resemble the Cell Danger Response. Absent the coordinating pulse of safety, autonomic systems stop functioning, or go rogue. Digestion stops working properly, and food that before nourished us can become toxic, just like the ATP. As this process unfolds, the immune system gets involved, pathogens are no longer deflected, co-occuring infections flare, and on and on, creating and intensifying the conditions for complex chronic illness.

At the end of our call Bob said, *I want to introduce you to a colleague of mine who is very gifted at treating complex chronic illness.*

Amazing, I said. *Does he live in the United States?*

It's a little town in Northern California, Bob said. *I think it is called San Rafael.*

That's funny, I said. Because I live in San Rafael. And that was how I met Dr. Eric Gordon.

02- TAKE TWO

Eric and I zoomed shortly after Bob's introduction, and met face-to-face for the first time on a spring afternoon in Nicasio, California, where I steward a forest. Meeting someone in a forest for the first time is great, because there is no clock on the wall. You sit outside together, the light filters through the trees and slowly changes as the sun makes its way across the sky, the birds sing, nature does its thing and you get to know someone outside of the tight strictures of the daily calendar that tells us we have a meeting at the top of the hour. Eric and I proceeded to have a series of conversations, about wellbeing and illness, about the Autonomic Nervous System and the immune system, about the difference between indigenous cosmovisions and modern cosmovisions, and then he started referring patients to me.

I think he would probably agree that this was not a great experience for either of us. Initially, Eric didn't know how to explain to his patients what I was doing, which created a situation where they would arrive and think we were having a long conversation when I was, in fact, taking precise histories and working with them autonomically. Sometimes a couple of hours into this, they would ask me when we were going to start, at which point they would be surprised to learn that they had already been paying my consultation rate for several hours. Not ideal. For me there was another problem, which is that Eric's patients were all very autonomically unwell. Because the way that I diagnose is largely felt, being around this level of autonomic dysregulation tended to make me feel sick for 24 hours after meeting with one of his patients. This had deleterious effects on my own sleep and general wellbeing. We did this for a few months before I stepped back. And when I stepped back I realized the thing that is the reason that I have written this book. I didn't really have to do autonomic diagnostics on Eric's patients because all of them presented with a common autonomic baseline.

There were individual variations in how they were sick, by which I mean the specific diagnosis (e.g., ME/CFS, Long COVID, Mast Cell Activation Syndrome, etc.), and the types of co-infections that most of them had (e.g., mold, Lyme Disease, etc.). But what all of them had in common were Autonomic Nervous Systems that had been pushed into, and were resistant to shifting out of, various formulations of lifethreat response. Some of these patients had this response blended with fight, some with flight, and some with sociality creating 'appease' or 'placating' autonomic states, but the common denominator for all was this shutdown response.

The second thing that all of them had in common was that there was not an immediate response to autonomic intervention, even if the intervention was appropriate. As in the Cell Danger Response, people in conditions of complex chronic illness were actually not sensitive to signals of safety from the Central Nervous System. Which is to say that, as distinct from a broad swath of people dealing with other kinds of stress-related issues, helping the nervous system detect safety was not enough to shift their autonomic baselines in real-time. The feedback loops from chronic lifethreat had simply moved other physiological systems too far in the direction of dysregulation.

This was frustrating both to the patients, and to myself, because we are used to seeing fairly immediate responses to neurological intervention in our work. But an important common feature of complex chronic illness is that it typically develops over decades. No one who is severely chronically ill becomes so in a short period of time. Complex chronic illness develops slowly through feedback loops that shift autonomic and metabolic baselines over long stretches of time, until a person's center of gravity shifts across a threshold into profound illness. And in our experience, their healing likewise takes significant time.

About a year after this initial foray into collaboration, Eric interviewed me for a series he was putting together on chronic illness. In preparing for our conversation he read my book *Autonomic Compass: Finding Home in your Nervous System*, and when he came into the conversation had developed a clearer understanding about the lens through which we view well- and ill-being.

After this conversation it occurred to me that it would be useful to his patients, and to others with complex chronic illness, if I were to write up a straightforward account of how we view complex chronic illness through the lens of the Autonomic Nervous System, and therefore how someone with complex chronic illness might begin to think about the origin, progression, and eventual healing of their illness from the standpoint of the Autonomic Nervous System.

That is the handbook you are now reading ;)

This book is not a bunch of hacks, and it does not contain 'a 28 day plan for re-tuning your Vagus nerve' or recommendations about vagal nerve stimulators. Buying a vagus nerve stimulator without understanding Autonomics is like walking into a building that's on fire with a bucket of water, slowly pouring it over the temperature sensor of the thermostat, and walking back out again. Most people don't have a problem with their vagus. Your life is on fire. That's the problem.

What I would like to do here is teach you how to put out the fire in your life. Implementing what I am describing here will probably take years, but I guarantee you that it will take place much faster than how long it took you to become this sick.

I'm gonna talk to you like we are having a conversation, because that's the way that I roll. My name is Gabriel. I am a connection phenomenologist, and neural cartographer, and the Developer of Autonomics, which up-ends several hundred years of classical neurology, and teaches people how to grasp and move the deepest and most powerful levers that govern your moment-to-moment experience of wellbeing. I am the Founder of Hearth Science, and I have taught autonomic physiology internationally for the past decade. I led a global autonomic physiology study group for wellness professionals with five thousand members, have trained about twenty thousand wellness practitioners around the world, and the books and software platform that I architected have helped people in fifty countries internationally.

I am deeply expert in this terrain, but it is also quite personal for me. I recovered from complex chronic illness in my twenties and thirties, but come from a family where several other members have not. Complex chronic illness is, to a degree that is not generally recognized, relational. And this is because the Autonomic Nervous System, which is the neural architecture of the mindbody connection, governs the energy-processing templates that shape the way that we relate to one another. What this means is that the roots of most complex chronic illness are laid down in early childhood, when we are learning non-verbally how to relate to those around us: our family, our siblings, the social systems in which we are enmeshed. This learning is not cognitive at all. It is, rather, deeply felt. Primal: animal if you will.

It is often here, in early childhood, that the templates for our defensive responses get organized: how we defend ourselves against threat. And so this is where we will begin the business of attempting to understand complex chronic illness through an autonomic lens.

03- EARLY CHILDHOOD

Human beings are born hairless and helpless, and without the proper caregiving will simply die. The fact that you are reading this sentence means that someone did a whole lot of work to keep you alive. If you think broadly about the animal kingdom, the degree to which a human infant is helpless is rather remarkable. Reptiles hatch from eggs, and when they are born, typically their parents are long gone. They have to innately possess all of the capabilities required to survive from the moment they hatch. Even many other mammals are much more adept at survival than human infants. A baby horse can typically walk within five minutes of being born, whereas a human infant needs 12 months. From an evolutionary perspective, this is rather perplexing, until we recognize something interesting.

Other animals that have brains as complex as ours, and here I'm speaking about creatures with similar degrees of cortical enfolding, like whales and elephants, typically have a gestation period that is closer to two years. A blue whale gives birth 24 months after conception. An elephant gives birth 22 months after conception. The human brain and nervous system likewise require this kind of time period to develop, but the evolutionary paradox we face is that our heads are so large that if we were to be fully cooked inside of our mothers, our heads would be too enormous to make their way out of the birth canal and we would not succeed in being born.

Nature solves this problem in an elegant yet paradoxical way. Human infants can be conceived as having a 27-month gestation period. The first nine months of this take place in utero. The next 18 months of it take place in two phases outside of the womb. Anthropologist Ashley Montagu calls this 18-month period the "womb with a view." It is the most developmentally sensitive period of human life (after our foetal stage), because it is the time in which our sensory and autonomic neurology is being completed and myelinated.

From a neuro-developmental perspective, a human baby isn't really born until the fontanelles close. Fontanelles are the sort of skylights in the skull that allows the cranium to slightly compress during the birth process, so the head can make its way out of the birth canal. There are two fontanelles. One is toward the front of the skull, one is toward the back of the skull. The first fontanelle typically knits closed at around three months of age, the second around 18 months of age. This closure of the fontanelles is contemporaneous with the completion of the infant's foundational neurological wiring. One of the insights of our research is that the myelination of critical autonomic systems is not complete until this point. In indigenous and ancestral cultures around the world, for the first nine months of life the infant is typically carried on the body of a caregiver skin-to-skin. Often they are never placed on the ground. The baby is essentially given a *womb with a view*. They are in touch proximity with a regulated caregiver, and the cultures understood that this developmental period was so sensitive that keeping the baby regulated was a crucial part of building the baby's brain and nervous system in ways that were required for flourishing. For this reason, in intact ancestral cultures, many people will nurse the baby. The whole point is to keep the baby in an optimal range of arousal. This comes from a profound understanding that the baby is still being formed neurologically at nine months of age. There is typically a transition, around the time the baby begins crawling, and for the next nine months, through the development of walking, the baby is still kept close and monitored closely as they move through the final 9-month 'trimester'.

Modern civilization has categorically and catastrophically failed to understand the significance of this 18-month developmental period. But if we are going to set our examination of the root causes of chronic illness on a firm foundation, this is where we have to start.

04- BUMPER STICKERS

There's a bumper sticker that reads, "We are not human beings having a spiritual experience: we are spiritual beings having a human experience."

If I was going to rewrite this through an autonomic lens, I would say that we are not material beings having an energetic experience, we are energy beings having a material experience. I am fairly well aware that to someone who does not live in California, this sentence might sound a little bit New Age. But that's not what I mean at all. When I say energy, I'm talking about energy in the $E=MC^2$ sense of it. In the Einsteinian interconversion between matter and energy sense of the word. Your autonomic nervous system is the mechanism in the body that interconverts matter and energy: that translates the flows of energy that run through you into experiences that you can metabolize; or not. I didn't study infant development in school, and so I really had no idea how sensitive an infant nervous system was until my daughter was born. I remember her arrival vividly for a variety of reasons. One of them was the astonishing completeness of this tiny being who had suddenly arrived after nine months in my wife's belly. I remember holding her reverently in the room in the hospital where we were staying, and I remember watching her sleep. One of the things that I find remarkable about infants is their complete commitment to whatever they're doing. Whether it is smiling, or weeping, or pushing out a poop, the effort and the commitment are total. The activity engages their entire being: mind, body and spirit.

When my daughter was born, she was so sensitive that I watched her startle awake at the click of a camera shutter. When a shift nurse in a bad mood entered our room, she would begin to wail inconsolably. From the moment she arrived, she could absolutely sense the energetic temperature of anyone around her. If their energy was clear, loving, and congruent, she would respond to this immediately. If a person approached her who was angry, irritated, frightened, sad, or upset, my daughter was immediately inconsolable. It became totally obvious that she was transparently feeling whatever energies were around her. She was picking up on the vibes.

This was not something she had to learn. It had nothing to do with cognition at all. And she could not tune it out. She had no defenses against feeling the vibrations of any beings nearby.

I am bringing this up, because at one point *you* were that tiny being. And although I have met a lot of humans in my nearly 50 years, I've never met one who was born into a totally enlightened family. All of us come in with that level of sensitivity, and then we are dropped into what my friend Shai Lavie calls *the nightmare of the nuclear family*. The challenge we have as tiny, extremely sensitive beings, is that we are often being cared for by people who do not understand the degree to which we are permeable to their energies, and have likely themselves suffered lifetimes of under-care and stress. This is a really major civilization-wide problem.

In the book that I am co-authoring with Darcia Narvaez, PhD, the developer of the Evolved Nest, we explore what is required to restore human nature (*Restoring Human Nature*). Any enlightened society, we propose, would place at its very center the mother-infant dyad, and organize all societal activities around the preservation of that relationship. Because if you want to build flourishing humans, you have to create the neurological conditions for building human wellness from the time the baby is conceived moving forward.

Sadly, it's not hard to see that our current incarnation of civilization so-called is not attending to caring for that relationship at all. Mothers are not supported during pregnancy. And none of our social structures are designed to prioritize their well-being, or the well-being of the family after the child is born. Instead, what happens for most of us is that we are taken home to houses with stressed-out parents and siblings. In order not to die in these environments, we have to learn pretty young how to defend ourselves against the onslaught of energies in these environments. And so this is where most of us begin to learn the defensive autonomic responses that will accompany us for most of our lives.

The good news is that if you're reading this sentence, the strategies that you deployed worked. From the perspective of the Autonomic Nervous System, the primary objective is survival. So it is a non-trivial thing to congratulate yourself on that. The strategies that you developed succeeded in keeping you alive! Good for you.

Unfortunately, for many people, these strategies are pretty maladaptive. Especially if we get caught in them habitually. And if you're reading this book, I can pretty much guarantee you that at least some of your foundational defensive strategies laid the neurological groundwork for the chronic illness you are now experiencing.

05- SOUND ENGINEER

Before we get any deeper into the text, I need to explain to you how I see the Autonomic Nervous System. I need to give you a few metaphors so that you can hold it close at hand, and understand it less abstractly. Classical neurology divides your nervous system into a Central Nervous System, and a Peripheral Nervous System. The Central Nervous System contains your brain and spinal cord. The Peripheral system is everything that is branching off of that. That peripheral system contains two distinct nervous systems. One of them is the Somatic Nervous System, which controls voluntary muscle. When I reach down to pick up my cup of coffee, I am engaging the somatic nervous system. It is volitional, which means that I choose to move in a particular direction. I choose to pick up the cup, and bring it to my lips. Now I choose to swallow the beverage it contains. The other peripheral nervous system is the Autonomic Nervous System. That's the one that we're gonna focus on.

For most people who have ever heard of the Autonomic Nervous System, they associate it with automatic responses. One of the Autonomic Nervous System's primary jobs is to regulate the internal milieu, which is to say that it's doing all of the housekeeping functions in the body so that you don't have to think about them. This is the part of your nervous system that breathes your breath, beats your heart, digests your food. You'll notice that I'm not saying that you are the one who is beating your heart, breathing, or digesting your food, because it's truly not your ordinary sense of self that is doing these things. You could totally forget about them, and the Autonomic Nervous System will perform these functions in the background. So it's important from the outset to recognize that you have a distinct sort of autonomic self that is making decisions about how to run the body that is not the same as your ordinary sense of

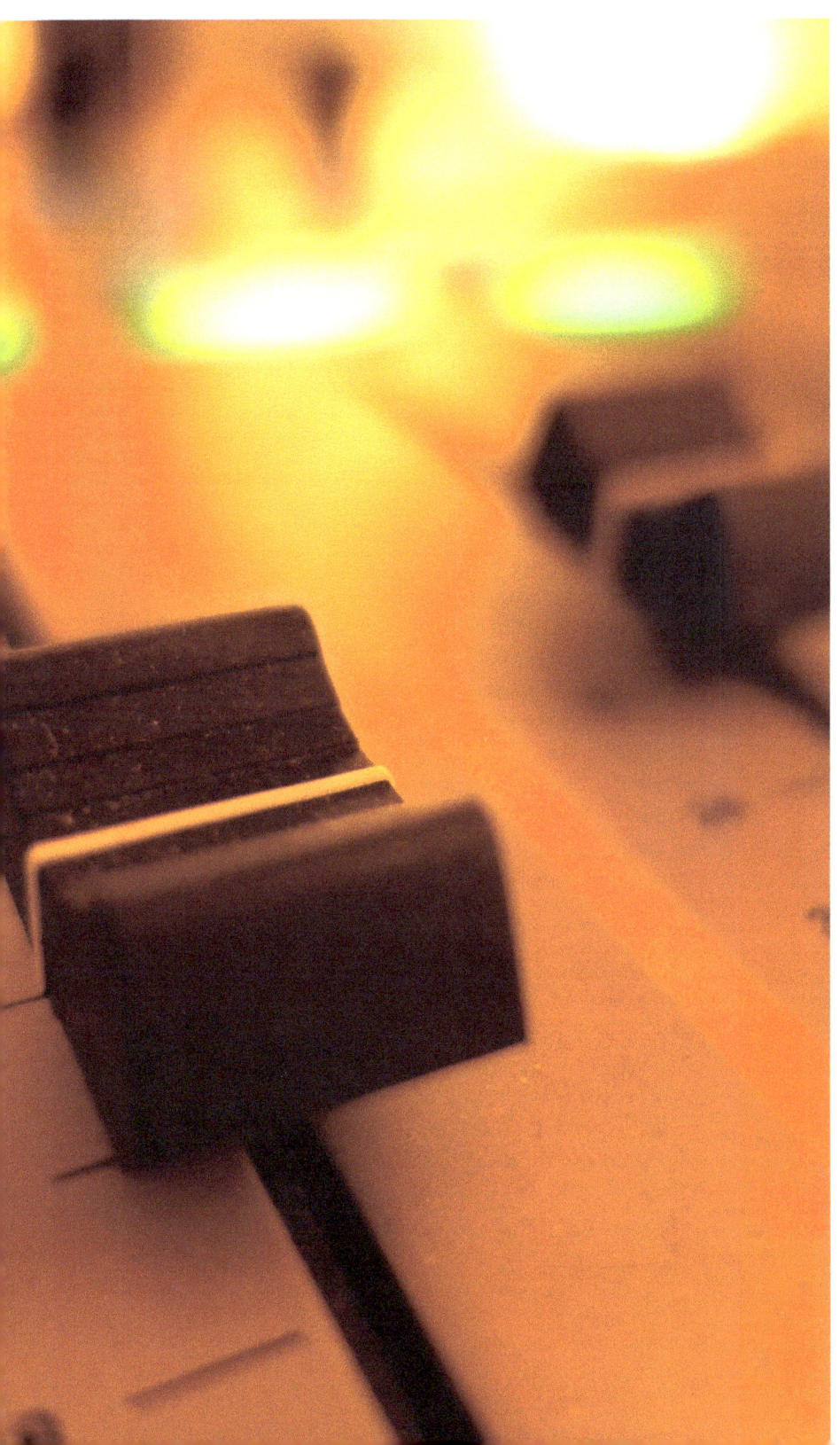

identity.

The second function of the Autonomic Nervous System, which is the particular purview of my expertise, involves the way that it re-tunes your body based on the moment-to-moment detection of safety, danger, or lifethreat. My mentor Stephen Porges, PhD, the developer of the Polyvagal Theory, coined the term *neuroception* to denote this particular discernment in the ANS.

I find it useful to think about the Autonomic Nervous System as a sound engineer. If you've ever been to a recording studio, or watched a studio session where musicians are recording an album, you'll notice that there is a room where the musicians are performing, and then off to the side there is a sound booth that contains a sound engineer. The engineer is typically looking at a console that has a bunch of knobs and dials on it, and their job is to adjust the balance of sound coming out of the instruments and the vocals in order to create the feel that the producers want for the tracks. It's pretty useful to think of your Autonomic Nervous System as this sound engineer. What the Autonomic Nervous System is doing, moment-to-moment, is optimizing the levels of your physiology in response to internal and external environmental cues. This modulation is happening much more dynamically than most people realize.

To simply transition from lying down to standing up and not pass out, you have to change a lot of physiological parameters in the body.[1] In order to stand up, heart rate has to increase moderately, and the contractile pressure has to increase. Tiny muscles have to tense in the base of the skull so that too much blood doesn't flow out of the brain and you don't get lightheaded. There are all kinds of reflexive fine-tuning autonomic adjustments made in the process of shifting from horizontal to vertical. Thankfully, we do not have to think about any of this stuff. Our Autonomic Nervous System is doing it for us.

---

1 Breakdowns in this coordinating capability of the ANS can present as orthostatic hypotension or Postural Orthostatic Tachycardia Syndrome (POTS).

And so, the sound engineer of the Autonomic Nervous System is the process that is dynamically recalibrating all of these levels in real-time. If we boil all of this down to its most distilled form, the genius of biology lies in our ability to conserve energy. And so what the Autonomic Nervous System has to decide in every moment is how the balance of energy in the body will be deployed. The primary calculus it uses to do this is survival-based. This is to say that if there is anything in our internal or external environment that is a threat to our survival, the vast majority of our energy resources will be deployed to address that specifically. In the absence of a threat, if we can downshift those defensive systems, we have reservoirs of energy available for life-affirmative processes. The long story of our evolutionary histories, however, is that there is a lot of dangerous shit in the world. And when that dangerous shit is happening, the sound engineers of the Autonomic Nervous System are prioritizing our survival responses.

Something that's really important for you to understand at the beginning is the following: having our survival responses enduringly activated is fundamentally incompatible with well-being. If we spend more of our moments in survival states, we will inevitably become sick. It is simply too metabolically costly. The Autonomic Nervous System cannot chronically reside in detections of danger and lifethreat without you becoming ill.

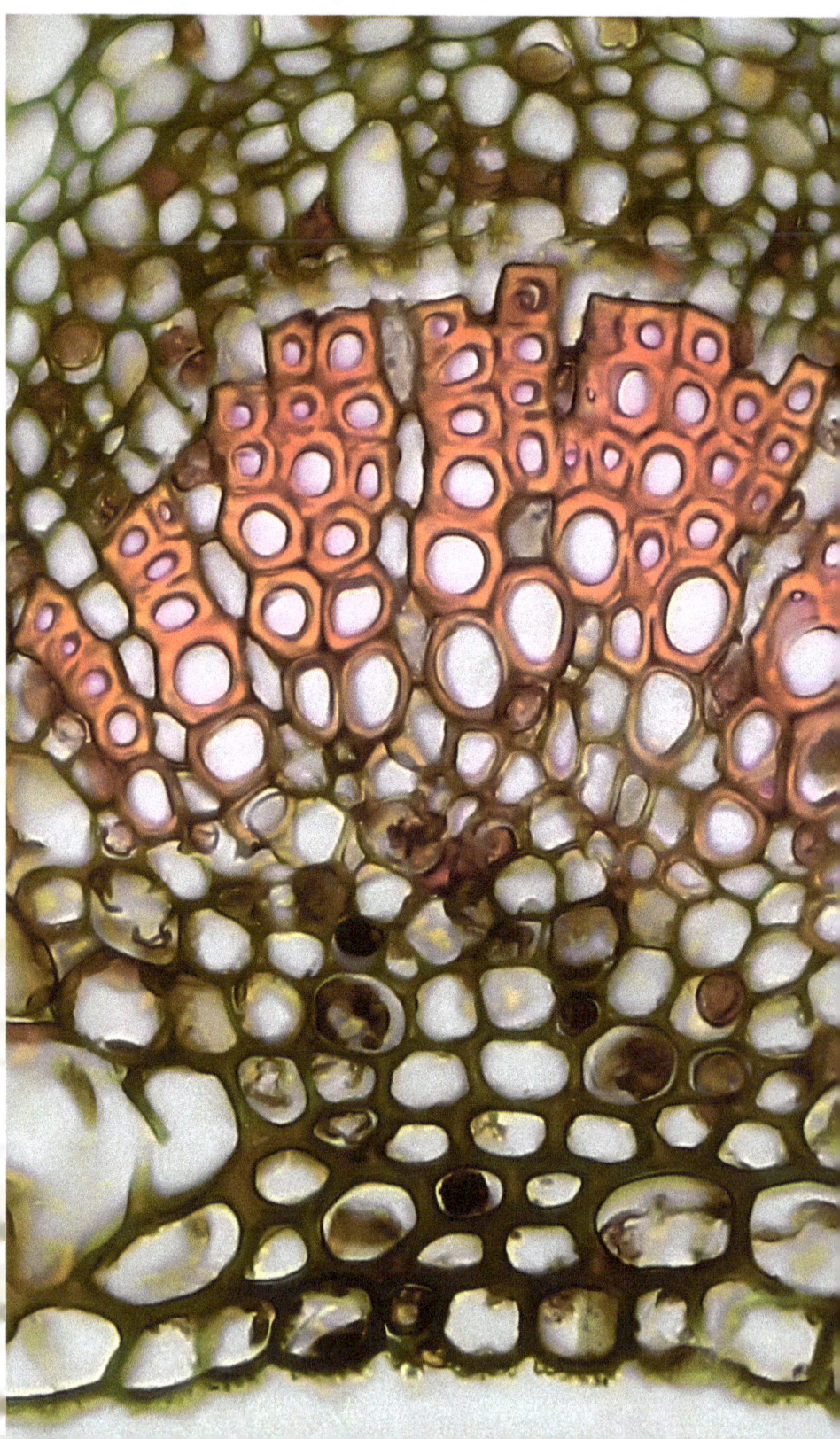

06- SYNTHESIS

OK, so now let's synthesize the last few chapters... We are these tiny highly sensitive beings. We come home after being born, not fully baked (not even close), and most of us end up in a house with a bunch of dangerously stressed-out monkeys.

The tiny sound engineers in our Autonomic Nervous System, acutely aware of both safety and threat, are tasked with helping us survive, and getting our needs met. If we can be startled awake by the click of a camera shutter, and burst into tears when a nurse who is unhappy enters the room, you can be pretty damn sure that we notice if people around us are calm and at ease, or screaming their heads off.

Most people who are stressed-out around a crying baby do not have the wherewithal to realize that it's probable that the baby is crying because of them. The next time you find yourself holding a baby who is crying, you might experiment with seeing what happens if you can bring yourself into a state of regulation. Often, the baby will immediately settle. This is not to say that there are not plenty of times when the baby is crying because it's hungry, or hot or cold, or has gas: it is rather to note that babies have almost no boundary, and are extremely sensitive to the energy of others.

And so that baby, who is you, ends up in the house that you were born into, having to navigate the energy landscape of a number of other stressed out human monkeys, while shit happens. And guess what: this is how you begin to develop and wire defensive autonomic states. For many people, this is when the pathway to developing complex chronic illness begins.

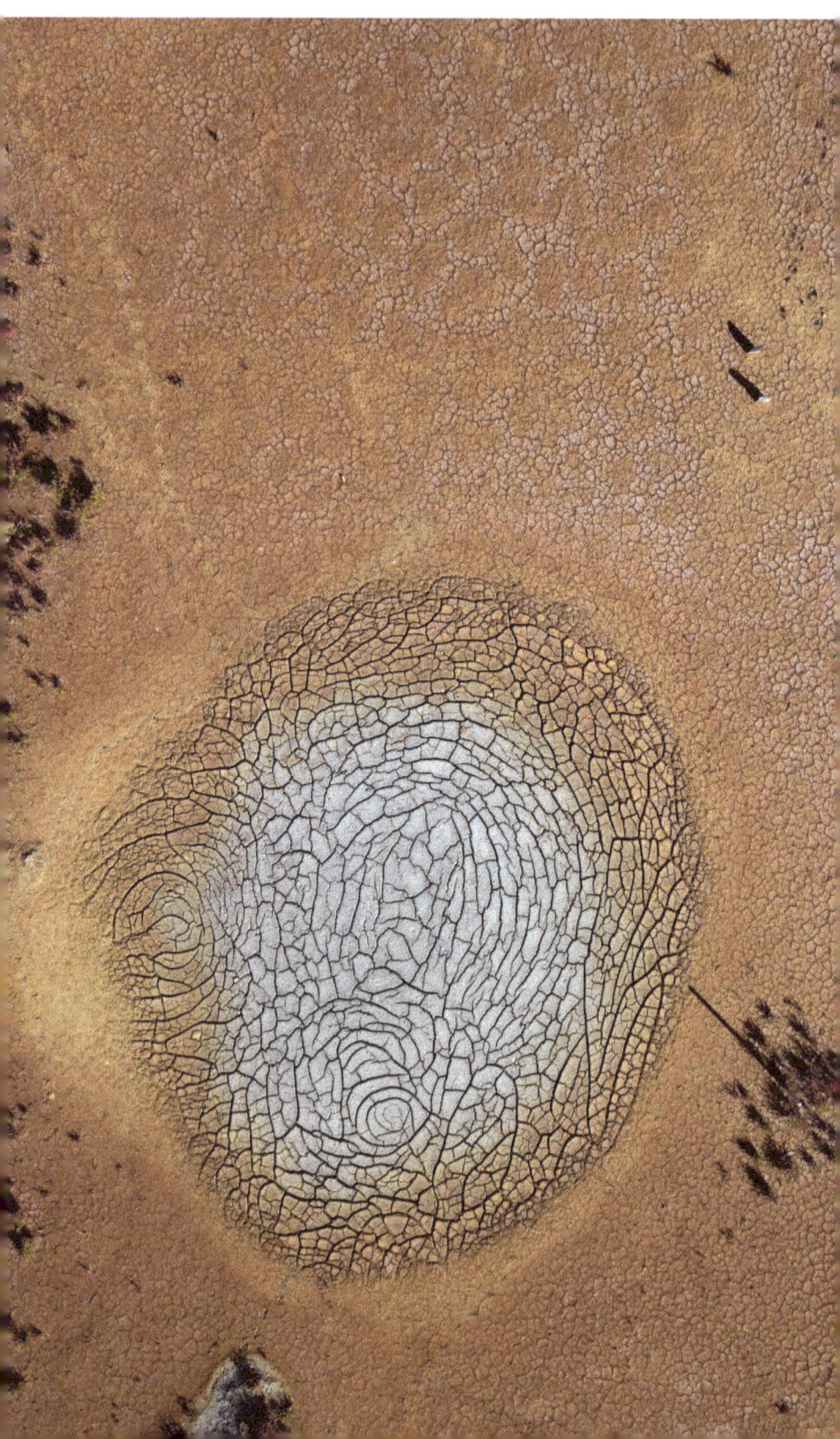

07- ACES

When I started Hearth Science, our very first client was a woman named Dr. Nadine Burke, who was at the time the Medical Director of a pediatric clinic in the Bayview/ Hunter's Point neighborhood of San Francisco. Nadine, who would go on to become the First Surgeon General of California under Gavin Newsom, is a protégé of Dr. Vincent Felitti, the Co-Principal Investigator of the Adverse Childhood Experiences study, which is one of the most significant epidemiological studies of trauma ever conducted. At the time the study was implemented, Dr. Felitti was the Chair of Preventive Medicine for the Southern California branch of Kaiser Permanente in San Diego. He was running several preventive medicine programs, including an obesity clinic, and a smoking cessation program.

Twenty-something years later, when I would interview him for a masterclass series on Connection Science that I was hosting, he would distill the insight that catalyzed the ACES study down into one of the most memorable phrases I've ever heard a physician utter. What Felitti began to suspect, was that, "The problems that we found ourselves treating in public health *were often the patient's solution to a much deeper problem that we could not see.*" By example, Felitti shared information with us about a couple of the cases that had catalyzed the study. One of them was a woman who had enrolled in the obesity clinic, and succeeded in losing about 200 pounds in a little over a year. He had been astonished: he did not know it was possible for a human being to lose weight that quickly. What then happened, however, was that the woman put all of the weight back on in less time than it had taken her to lose it. The catalyst for this sudden weight gain was her being approached and sexually propositioned by a colleague at work. What Felitti began to suspect was that the woman's weight was a costly yet effective strategy to prevent her from garnering sexual attention, which recalled to her the unmanageable trauma of a history of childhood sexual abuse. *Her obesity was actually not the problem, but rather the costly solution to a deeper problem that they could not see.* What Felitti began to recognize was that in successfully treating the obesity, or the tobacco use, he was actually taking away his patient's primary coping strategy.

At a conference detailing the results of some of his work in preventive medicine, Felitti met Robert Anda, an epidemiologist at the Centers for Disease Control in Atlanta. Together, they conceived the study that would become known as the Adverse Childhood Experiences study. In the study, Felitti integrated ten questions about categories of early childhood abuse and neglect into an adult health screening questionnaire administered to patients at Kaiser in San Diego. By the time the study was complete, they had gathered data from 17,421 adults. The picture the study painted was stark. Two thirds of an adult population at a private pay insurer in Southern California had exposure to at least one Adverse Childhood Experience.

Furthermore, Felitti found a graded dose-response relationship between the incidents of early adversity, and the development of all categories of disease later in life, across both physical and mental health domains. The average age of respondents in the study was 57 years old, and most people were reporting on experiences that had occurred nearly 50 years prior. What the study showed us definitively was that the impacts of early childhood adversity endure. We are told that time heals all wounds, but in the case of traumatic exposures this is simply not true.

The reason that this is not true is that trauma creates enduring changes in our neurobiological setpoints. Stress is accumulated, and locked into the body through neurological and chemical alterations. If these are not addressed– if we cannot find a way to get back to neurological baselines, and clear the accumulated loads and chemistry, the body and mind are permanently functionally altered.

Because of the way that the study was organized and framed, distinctions were not made between the types of stress responses that a child elicited in response to an early adverse experience. Yet what we know from our study of autonomic physiology is that two people can experience the same event, and respond to it in very different ways, by evoking completely different defensive survival responses. Some people love public speaking, and others are terrified of it. Two siblings can be in the room with parents who are arguing, have different interpretations of what happened, and be impacted in totally different ways. Our experience of events is highly contextual, and contingent upon our own nervous systems. This is why we often say in the field of trauma healing that *trauma is in the nervous system, not the event.*

If we could re-author the ACES study with the use of wearable autonomic diagnostic tracking tools that happened to be on the children at the time of their exposure to adverse experiences, we could more successfully quantify the types of allostatic loads that various exposures to adversity have on the human body. Because overwhelming experiences put us into autonomic survival responses, and because these responses re-tune the body in characteristic ways, causing us to accumulate quantifiable levels of stress, a more algorithmically sophisticated version of the study could show us the particular ways that early events impact a specific child going forward. Yet Felitti's study was slightly more anecdotal. There was no biometric measurement around the inciting incidents.

Yet what still became patently obvious was that a much larger percentage of the population than previously recognized had exposure to early traumatic events, and their impacts were enduring throughout the lifespan. This is important for us to understand when we are thinking about chronic illness through an autonomic lens, because it validates the notion that the roots of these kinds of diseases often reach back to early childhood.

Again, something that's foundational to thinking about chronic illness through an autonomic lens is likewise the recognition that the most important determinant of illness is not the event– it's not specifically what happened– it is how our particular autonomic nervous system responded to that overwhelming experience. This might seem counter-intuitive at first, especially because most of us are pretty identified with our stories about what has happened in our lives, and why we have become the way that we are. But if we're going to dig down to the layers at which transformation can happen, it is important for us to understand the degree to which our focus should be on the way that the autonomic sound engineer has altered or re-tuned our nervous system, more than the specific music that was playing when this happened. Talk therapy is wonderful, and having insights about our own histories is very important, but neither of them moves the needle on the actual physiological processing of overwhelming experience, and this is where you want the needle to move if you are seeking healing.

Take a moment and think about the ways that various people you know might respond to the same stressor in different ways. I can think of situations where something stressful has happened in the life of my family, and it made me angry, made my wife anxious, and made my daughter sad. All of these responses are autonomic, and all of them are valid responses to threat. Both my wife's response and my own are undergirded by what traditional neurology calls the Sympathetic Nervous System. They also primarily involve the biochemistries of adrenaline and cortisol. But my fight response, whose emotional correlate is anger, and which is designed to directly confront a threat, feels very different than my wife's flight response, whose emotional correlate is fear, and whose purpose is to get her away from a threat. These are both distinct from my daughter's response, which involves a different autonomic pathway, is more concerned with becoming socially invisible, and is mediated by the biochemistries of endogenous opioids.

I'm not placing any particular value judgment on one response or the other: I'm just noticing that these are three different adaptive responses to a threat with entirely different felt qualities (anger, anxiety, sadness) undergirded by differing neurology and neurochemistry. Beyond our three responses, a fourth person might respond by appeasing, and a fifth by placating.

Part of developing autonomic fluency is knowing how our particular nervous systems respond to stressful events. If you have developed complex chronic illness, we already know something about this, because these kind of illnesses only develop when a person habitually responds to stressors with a specific subset of autonomic defensive responses.

What I'd like you to take away from this chapter on ACES is the awareness that early experiences of adversity that push the Autonomic Nervous System into defensive states have enduring impacts on well-being over the lifespan. In addition, the specific autonomic energy processing templates that our nervous system evoked to respond to threats govern the kind of illness that we may develop over time. Beginning to understand why our specific autonomic nervous systems respond to survival threats the way that they do is the first step in moving towards transforming these responses.

08- THE FIGHT-FLIGHT RESPONSES

Over the past six years, the firm I direct has assembled either the first, second, or third largest dataset on the relationship between autonomic state and the etiology of disease in the world. In working autonomically with clients in fifty countries, we have assembled a map of the thirteen most common autonomic states, as well as a map of the way that the defensive survival responses, if they become chronic and enduring, undergird various disease processes.

The common denominator of all chronic illness is the movement of the body into lifethreat states.

When we are threatened, the body has two primary autonomic options in responding. The first response, which is what most people think of when they think about stress, involves the fight-or-flight pathways. Fight-or-flight responses are mobilization responses, which means that the body wants to move in responding to the threat. These responses make primary use of the vertebrate Movement System, known in traditional neurology as the Sympathetic Nervous System. This system is as ancient as the vertebrate body plan, and includes the kind of reflex arcs that are designed to move our bodies away from danger, or fight it off. *It is important to understand that fight-or-flight responses are movement-based.* These responses are also polarizing, which means that part of their function is to help us discern, at a biological level, who is with us, and who is against us.

In the moment when the fight response turns on, we determine that whomever we are getting ready to fight is a *them*, not an *us*. We set a boundary, and the person toward whom our fight energy is directed is outside of it. We do not experience empathy towards them: they no longer fall within our circle of care. In this sense, fight-or-flight responses are *boundary-setting* responses.

These two attributes: *mobilized*, and *polarized*, are the embodied signatures of fight-flight responses. These responses are undergirded by the biochemistries of adrenaline[1] and cortisol. A surge of adrenaline is what you feel when you drink a double espresso. Adrenaline increases our heart rate, accelerates our breathing, raises our blood pressure, elevates our blood sugar levels, and focuses our gaze, while enhancing alertness and reducing pain sensitivity. This is a potent combination of effects. Cortisol complements the role of adrenaline by also increasing the bio-availability of sugar in the blood, in tandem with suppressing the immune system (it is anti-inflammatory), and tightening the muscles.

AUTONOMIC AWARENESS PRACTICE: NOTICING THE EMBODIED SIGNATURE OF THE FIGHT RESPONSE

With the goal of increasing your own autonomic awareness, take a moment to allow yourself to register the physical and emotional responses that accompany the fight-flight responses.

Think about how it feels when you shift into a mode where you want to fight someone or something (and it doesn't have to be a physical fight, mind you. This could be true of an argument, or fighting something legally, or politically, etc.) The heart beats faster, you become more alert, the body prepares for action, et cetera. Notice that the emotional correlate of this response is anger. Notice how hard it is to feel empathy for someone or something you've decided you are going to fight.

Take a moment to remember a time when you've gone into a fight response. Choose something that is of moderate intensity, by which I mean an event that is not tiny (fighting over a paperclip), but is not enormous (fighting in a war).

---

1 I'm using the British version of the name of the hormone/neurotransmitter here, because it is used more commonly, but this is the same substance as epinepherine.

- How can you tell, in your body, that you are in a fight response?
- What does the body feel like at a muscular level? What is the level of tension?
- Many people feel the energy of the fight response in their hands and arms. Is that true for you?
- How is your breathing?
- How is your heartrate?
- What is your vision doing?
- How is your attention moving?
- What is the emotional tone you notice?
- What are your thoughts like?
- What else do you notice about how your attention resides in your body and mind?
- What are the personal signatures for you that allow you to notice that you are having a fight response?

I realize that some of the questions above might seem obvious to you, but one of the things that continues to fascinate me, having studied the Autonomic Nervous System for decades, is the degree to which autonomic changes often happen outside of our conscious awareness. Remember that the part of ourselves that is making autonomic determinations (the sound engineer) is not our ordinary sense of self.

Often the thing that triggers an autonomic response is not something that we are fully aware of. We can shift autonomically because we start ruminating on a disturbing experience, or because someone cuts us off in traffic. The degree to which we are present with and recognize this shift determines how able we are to do anything about it. Often I come to realize I have shifted into a fight response by the number of f-bombs that are arising in my internal dialogue. If I find myself, in my own private mind going, "F*ck this, f*ck that," it's a pretty clear signal to me that I've moved into a defensive fight response.

A corollary to this effect is that often we have already taken steps to self-soothe or self-medicate in response to an autonomic trigger before we realize that we have been triggered. Stress-eating is a simple example of this. Sometimes I realize I am feeling stressed because I notice that there is chocolate in my hand. If I track back to the moment I started craving chocolate, I can often get back to the autonomic triggering event. Does that make sense? Sometimes we can realize that we have shifted autonomically because we have started engaging a coping mechanism. This is what Felitti was pointing out.

Knowing the autonomic signature of a shift into a defensive response in your own body is the first crucial awareness building step that starts to give your some optionality and agency around responding. You might not find yourself reaching for chocolate, but perhaps instead it is a cigarette. Nicotine has, for example, extraordinary anti-anxiety properties. For someone whose go-to stress response is flight, nicotine is a costly yet effective solution to moving into a defensive autonomic response. Again, the problem is not the cigarettes: they are the solution. But it is hard to do anything about the habit if we cannot feel the underlying shift into distress that ignites the craving, which is the quasi-automatic coping strategy that engages in response to a change in this autonomic baseline.

I'd also like to encourage you to notice if it is hard for you to allow yourself to feel the energy of the fight response. For many people with chronic illness, the very idea of the fight response is frightening, which is to say that it is not on the menu of autonomic responses available. Some of us learned early in life that engaging in a fight response when we were under threat was not ok. The internalized prohibition against fight may be so deep that it simply feels impossible for us to generate the energies of fight. The prohibition against it may be moral: e.g., if we fight we are a bad person. Or it may simply be learned from growing up in environments where, for example, one of our parents was violent, and if we fought back things went worse for us. It could also be the case that we learned, based on our social location (e.g., gender, race, religion, nationality, etc.,) that engaging in a fight response was simply too dangerous. If our Autonomic Nervous Systems learn that a defensive response may get us killed, it likely comes off the menu of possible responses. If you recognize that the fight response is not on your menu, simply notice that: we'll come back to this later. Don't judge it at all, rather recognize that this is crucial information that will be important to your healing journey going forward.

AUTONOMIC AWARENESS PRACTICE: NOTICING THE EMBODIED SIGNATURE OF THE FLIGHT RESPONSE

Let's try the same kind of exercise with the flight response.

Think about how it feels when you shift into a mode where you want to flee someone or something. Notice that the emotional correlate of this response is fear.

Take a moment to remember a time when you've gone into a flight response. Choose something that is of moderate intensity, by which I mean an event that is not tiny (fleeing from the wind), but is not enormous (fleeing a natural disaster).

- How can you tell, in your body, that you are in a flight response?
- What does the body feel like at a muscular level? What is the level of tension?
- Many people feel the energy of the flight response in their legs and feet. Is that true for you?
- How is your breathing?
- How is your heartrate?
- What is your vision doing?
- How is your attention moving?
- What is the emotional tone you notice?
- What are your thoughts like?
- What else do you notice about how your attention resides in your body and mind?
- What are the personal signatures for you that allow you to notice that you are having a flight response?

Notice also whether is feels easier for you to recall and imagine having a fight response versus having a flight response. This is in fact very valuable information about your particular Autonomic Nervous System. Notice as well if it is difficult for you to summon the energies of flight. Again, some people find this very hard. They might not be able to imagine themselves getting away successfully. Again, even if it is uncomfortable to notice this about yourself, it is extremely valuable information. Part of our goal in developing autonomic fluency is to get all of the health-creating responses back on the menu, and all of the defensive responses back on the menu. We want to have response flexibility so that we do not automatically fall back into a single defensive response. If you find that it is difficult for you to feel the flight response in the body, bookmark this. We will come back to this later in the chapter focused on reclaiming defensive responses.

Let's imagine that you have gone out to dinner with two friends in the city, and that afterwards you are going to see a concert. The restaurant is a few blocks from the concert venue, and after dinner you are now walking with your friends up the street to see the show. You can see the marquis of the theatre a few blocks up. You and your friends are walking together, talking and laughing. Now imagine that out of the corner of your eye you notice someone approaching you diagonally from the opposite side of the street, a couple of hundred feet away. The person is staggering a little: they look unsteady. It is hard to tell if they are drunk, on drugs, or wounded. It is also hard to tell if they just happen to be walking vaguely in your direction, or they are actually approaching you on purpose. Imagine that you can feel your level of arousal begin to rise.

What you might do— what many humans in this situation might do— is to offer a social engagement cue to this person and see if they respond. If the person is looking at you, you might do this by greeting them, or giving them a little head nod, or asking if they are ok. If the person gives you any sort of a reciprocal response, anything to let your Autonomic Nervous System know that you are not in danger, your arousal level may drop back down. But if not, it is likely that you will move in the direction of a defensive response.

Depending on your history, social location, and embodied assessment of the danger, you may move into a fight-flight response, or a shutdown response. As you do this, the body dramatically re-tunes. You would find it suddenly difficult to hear your friends as your ears re-tune away from the midrange of human vocalization to focalize predator signals, which tend to be lower frequency. Your attention would tend to fixate on the threat, making it hard to look away from this approaching person. The sound engineer in the Autonomic Nervous System is moving the levers and dials to keep you alive in a dangerous world. If you imagine this situation, and consider what your body would be most likely to do in response, it may give you a window into your habitual response to threat. Some people are likely to get combative, some get ready to run, and some people feel immobilized, frozen on the spot. Some people might try to appease the stranger, or placate them. All of this can come into focus for you simply by imagining this scenario. This gives you a great deal of information about how your Autonomic Nervous System is pre-conditioned by your life experiences.

Again, I am placing no value judgement on the response. I haven't told you the gender of the person approaching, their age, their race, or any other contexual information: I'm letting your own Autonomic Nervous System fill all of those blanks in, which I presume it has already done. I'm simply giving you an empty threat signal, and letting you notice how your ANS fills in the sketch and responds.

People who have not studied autonomic physiology are often astonished by the severity with which the autonomic nervous system can re-tune our minds and bodies in the presence of threat. It is deeply unfortunate that autonomic fluency is not taught in elementary school. As we begin to understand the ferocity of these responses, and the magnitude of alteration they can make to the way our bodies work, how we feel, how we think, how we interpret the world around us, and how we behave, it renders a lot of extreme and otherwise incomprehensible behavior obvious. People who escalate rapidly into violent high-intensity responses are often people who experience extreme lack of safety.

When we move from a neuroception of safety, to a neuroception of danger, we experience fundamental perceptual changes. The way that our eyes work changes completely, because in the presence of a threat, our optical systems are co-opted by our survival responses. This means that there is sudden visual salience given to potential threats. This can feel as if our eyes are now suddenly searching for all potential sources of danger, and become easily fixated on possible threats. We might, if we shift into a defensive response in a grocery store, for example, suddenly find our eyes searching for exits. The way that our hearing works changes. When we feel safe enough to become available, our middle ear selectively tunes to the prosody of the human voice, which is in a vocal mid-range. Under threat, however, the middle ear re-tunes, and now what we hear are the deep bass frequencies of predators. These changes are not in our minds, they are not psychological, they are not some kind of placebo effect. These are physiological changes in the fundamental control settings of our bodily perceptual systems. Adjustments to the knobs and levers of our deep nervous system.

In tandem with these sensory changes, the body, during a threat response, downshifts the systems that are not essential to ensuring our survival. What this means at a practical level is that many of the life-sustaining and supporting activities that are associated with states of resting and restoration get turned off. And with specific regard to chronic illness, one of the most important systems that is always down-regulated in stress responses is our digestion.

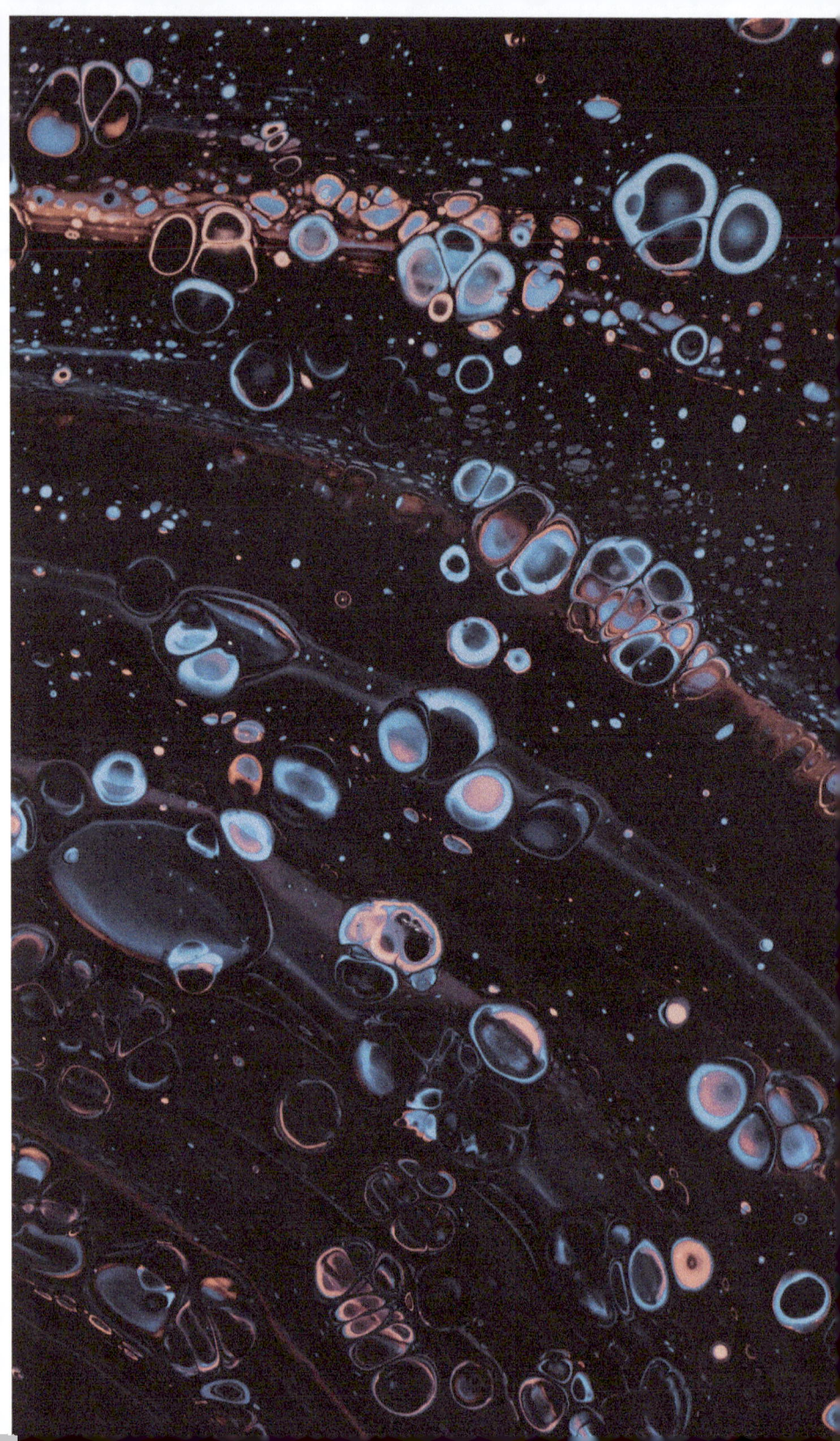

09- DIGESTIVE DIFFICULTIES AND THE LIFE-THREAT RESPONSE

The incidence of gastro-intestinal disease is steadily increasing globally.[1] This is partly a function of the global introduction of genetically modified foodstuffs (GMOs), but it is even more a reflection of greater and greater swaths of humanity moving increasingly into states of chronic and non-resolving stress response.

Because from the immediate perspective of survival, digestion is not an essential function, digestive processes are systematically down-regulated during a stress response. The stress response is evolutionarily designed to be rapid in onset, and rapid in resolving, but in our modern circumstances, which tend to lack the ancestral village and the neurological inputs of the Living World, it increasingly fails to resolve, which leaves people in a state where digestion can be compromised enduringly. I'm going to lay out the neurobiological sequelae of this problem in a moment, but I first would like to distinguish between the fight-flight responses, and the shutdown responses, with respect to the ways that they impact digestion.

While both responses have adverse impacts on digestion, the impacts of lifethreat responses are particularly problematic and severe. Let's start with a little bit of a primer on the shutdown response. We've talked about fight-or-flight. And in the situation that we described where we were going to see a concert with a friend, and were approached by someone whose motives we could not interpret, we examined the way that a fight-or-flight response might alter our physiology. In polyvagally-informed trauma training, the shutdown response is viewed as the survival response of last resort. Often it is taught as the

---

1 *Increasing Incidence and Prevalence of the Inflammatory Bowel Diseases With Time, Based on Systematic Review*
https://www.sciencedirect.com/science/article/abs/pii/S0016508511013783

response that happens when fight-or-flight strategies fail. If, for example, we try to fight something off, and are not successful, then try to flee and are not successful, we will move into a shutdown response as a last resort.

What I would like to assert categorically, based on 15 years of our own research and clinical work in this area, is that most people, by the time they are adults, if the shutdown response is a habitual response to threat, may entirely skip going through fight-or-flight responses when there is a stressor, and simply move straight into shutdown. If our bodies learned to move into shutdown during childhood, or as the result of a serious traumatic injury, and this autonomic state is something that has happened previously, it becomes more likely to happen again.[2] The lifethreat response is self-reinforcing in this regard, which is to say that once it enters the behavioral repertoire, it is more likely to repeat.

What this means functionally, is that by the time a person is a grown-up, their nervous system is no longer a blank slate. Approached by an ambiguous threat, if the shutdown response is a go-to response, the system is just as likely to go directly to this response as to move through a progression in its direction. *The more time we spend in any autonomic response, the more gravity it has to pull on our system in the event of a threat.*

The shutdown response is the evolutionarily oldest and deepest survival response. Its neurological mechanism is a 500-millionyear-old diving reflex, and an organism uses the response to get to safety by radically dropping the metabolic rate and immobilizing. It is a response that allows us to become socially invisible. Whereas the fight-or-flight responses are mobilization responses, which means that they specifically involve motor movement, the shutdown response is neurologically characterized by immobilization. When the body moves into a shutdown response, the breathing slows dramatically, heartrate

---

2 Evocation of an autonomic defensive state is a function of neuroception, and the archived allostatic load affiliated with that state.

plummets, and the body immobilizes. The biochemistry undergirding this response is the release of endogenous opioids.

The body naturally produces an arsenal of endogenous opioids, including a class called enkephalins. These neuro-modulators selectively target the central pattern generators (CPGs) of the vertebrate Movement System, and when a person moves into a lifethreat response, this biochemistry takes our Movement System off-line.

It feels important to point out how the release of endogenous opioids makes us feel. Most people regularly ingest substances that mimic or increase the production of adrenaline. If you start your day with a cup of coffee, and do a before/after examination, e.g., how do you feel before drinking it; how do you feel after, you have a pretty clear sense of what adrenaline feels like. Yet most people lack a similar experiential analog for endogenous opioids, unless they've taken opioid painkillers at some point in their lives.

For pedagogical purposes then, I would like to point out that one of the active ingredients in most cough medicine, dextromethorphan, which is technically part of the chemical family of morphinans, binds to the same opioid receptors as enkephalins, and possesses both of their primary effects, which are to say that it is analgesic (painkilling) and dissociative. If you've ever taken cough medicine for a chest cold, or to clear congestion, you may have some memory of the specific ways that it can make you feel loopy, detached, disconnected from what is happening around you (these are the dissociative properties of the chemical). I have personally found myself hallucinating on Mucinex, which is one of the OTC cough medicines, another effect of the uptake of dextromethorphan by opioid receptors in the Central Nervous System. So if you need a tangible sense of how the specific release of enkephalins feels in the body, think about how you feel when you've taken cough medicine.

Earlier in the text, I explained that health-creating states have all three fundamental autonomic systems available and coordinated. When we shift into defensive survival responses, the Connection System is no longer available to us. In the fight-or-flight responses, we have two autonomic systems functionally available: the Movement System and the Grounding System. ***Shutdown responses are the only autonomic states where we have simply one autonomic system available.*** This system is the sub-diaphragmatic Grounding System, comprised of unmyelinated vagal circuitry in the guts.

In its lifethreat configuration, we might more accurately think of the system as the *Ungrounding System*, because what it does functionally is disconnect us from our roots. We literally stop being able to feel the ground under our feet.

When the body re-tunes into a lifethreat response, it brings digestion to a screeching halt. Because the response is essentially an ancient diving reflex, one of its primary manifestations is a fundamental inhibition on breath. As the breath slows, and the metabolic rate drops, the body begins to de-oxygenate.

Humans are able to successfully digest the range of foods we consume because our digestive system hosts a garden of microorganisms that aid in this process. Known as the gut microbiome, this garden of microscopic gut flora is responsible for helping us break down our foods, and also produces many of the micro-nutrients that we need. Like any garden, its health depends on a number of contextual factors. If you do any gardening at all, you know that most plants have very specific preferences for how much sunlight and water they need, as well as the soil attributes that they require in order to flourish. Your gut microbiome is no different. Moving into a stress response, and particularly a lifethreat response, radically alters the immediate environmental context for the gut microbiome.

Our digestive system is essentially a long segmented tube that winds from the mouth to the anus. The microbiome exists in distinct pockets along this tube, differentiated by the various

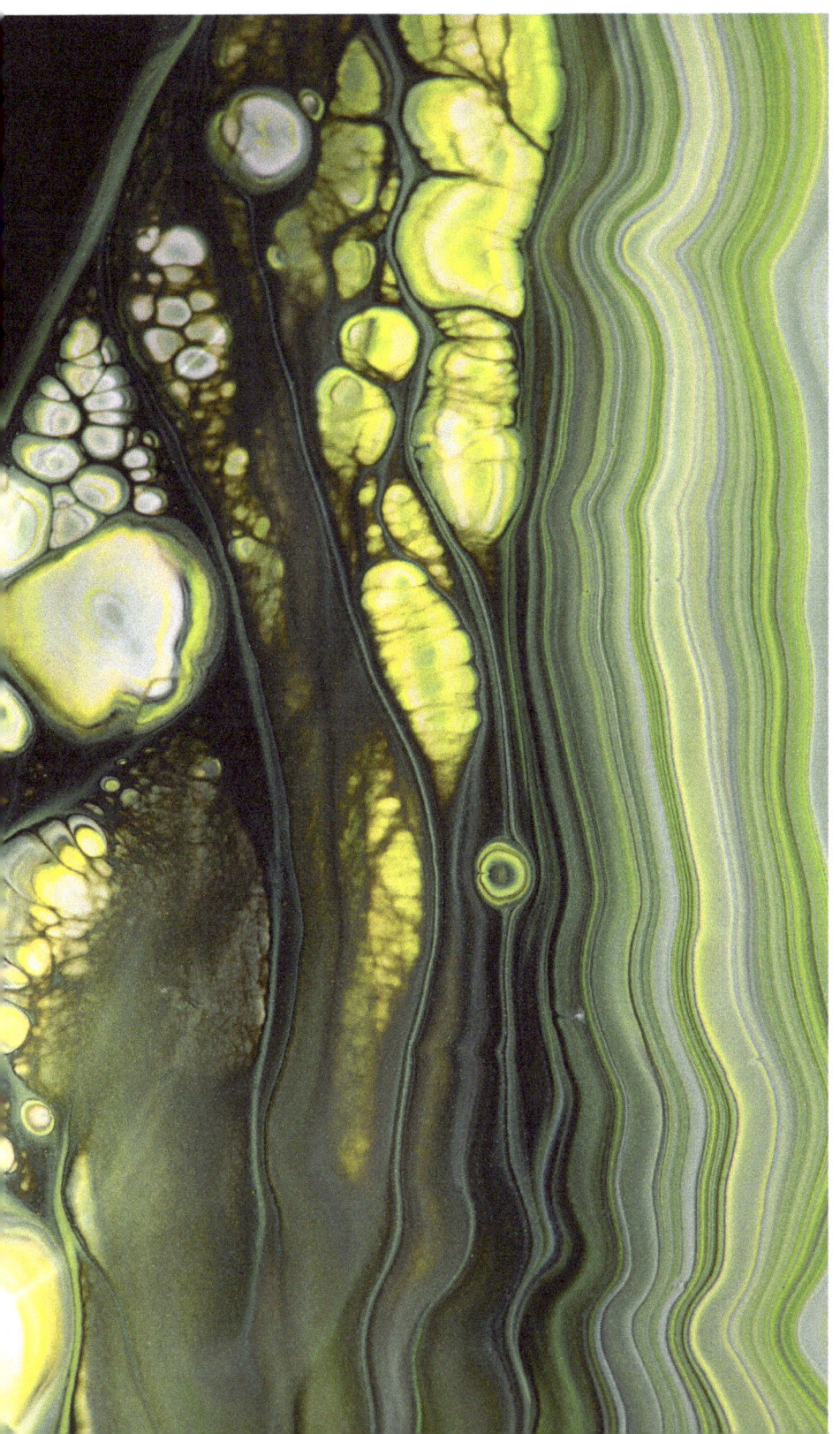

sphincters that separate the stomach from the small intestine from the large intestine. The tube is increasingly anaerobic as it goes deeper into our bodies. There is more oxygen in the stomach than in the small intestine, than in the large intestine. When we shift into a lifethreat response, and the breathing becomes inhibited, the entire system begins to deoxygenate. This changes the metabolic conditions of the entire digestive tube, and as a result begins to change the pH of these environments.

Furthermore, the stress response increases our metabolic demand for glucose. The brain in particular is very hungry for sugar. If levels of sugar in the blood fall beneath certain thresholds, we strongly crave sugar. Sugar has very specific effects on the microbiome. It is a preferred food for many of the micro-organisms that we do not wish to see proliferating, and it also has adverse impacts on our immune system. This combination of deoxygenation of the guts, which changes the pH balance, with a concomitant addition of sugar creates a situation where we tend to encourage micro-organisms that we do not want, and discourage the ones that we do, while disabling the immune system.

As toxic micro-organisms proliferate, they begin to excrete poisons. Effective digestion depends on the microvilli of the large intestine, where nutrients are absorbed into the bloodstream. Exposure to the toxic chemistry from these micro-organisms can begin to irritate the intestinal lining of the large intestine. As this happens, the tight junctions between epithelial cells begin to gap. This can effectuate the passage of molecules into the bloodstream that should not ordinarily enter it. If this happens, the immune system engages, because suddenly there are molecules escaping from the digestive system and entering the blood that should not be. Inflammatory cytokines are released. We began to develop what is commonly known as leaky gut. This is the predictable neurobiological sequelae of residing in a chronic and non-resolving lifethreat state. As this process progresses, it moves into varying flavors of inflammatory bowel disease (IBD).

10 - THE DIFFERENCE BETWEEN FREEZE AND SHUTDOWN

There are several discrete variants of the lifethreat response, the distinctions between which are not generally understood by the mainstream population. This is partly a result of confusion that has arisen from Dr. Peter Levine's work in Somatic Experiencing®, where the term 'freeze response' entered common parlance. Dr. Levine developed a naturalistic approach to the resolution of trauma, based in part on watching animals in the wild, with extraordinary efficacy in treating certain kinds of overwhelming experiences.

In his book *Waking the Tiger: Healing Trauma*, he utilizes the term 'freeze response' to speak about lifethreat responses as distinct from fight-or-flight. This notion of freeze is metaphorically accurate, as it conveys the qualities of immobility that are characteristic of lifethreat responses. Speaking more technically, however, with a broader understanding of the fully differentiated range of autonomic lifethreat responses, we need to distinguish this freeze response from a pure shutdown response. What is the difference between the two?

A freeze response is technically called *tonic immobility*. This is the kind of phenomenon observed when someone sees a deer in headlights. In a tonic immobility response, there is both immobilization and muscle rigidity. Muscle rigidity is a function of the vertebrate Movement System. So at a technical level, the freeze response is actually a combination of shutdown and sympathetic responses. This is distinct from a pure lifethreat response, which does not have access to the Movement System at all, and therefore does not have muscular rigidity. In a pure shutdown response, there is no muscle tone. In its most complete presentation, the person will simply pass out.

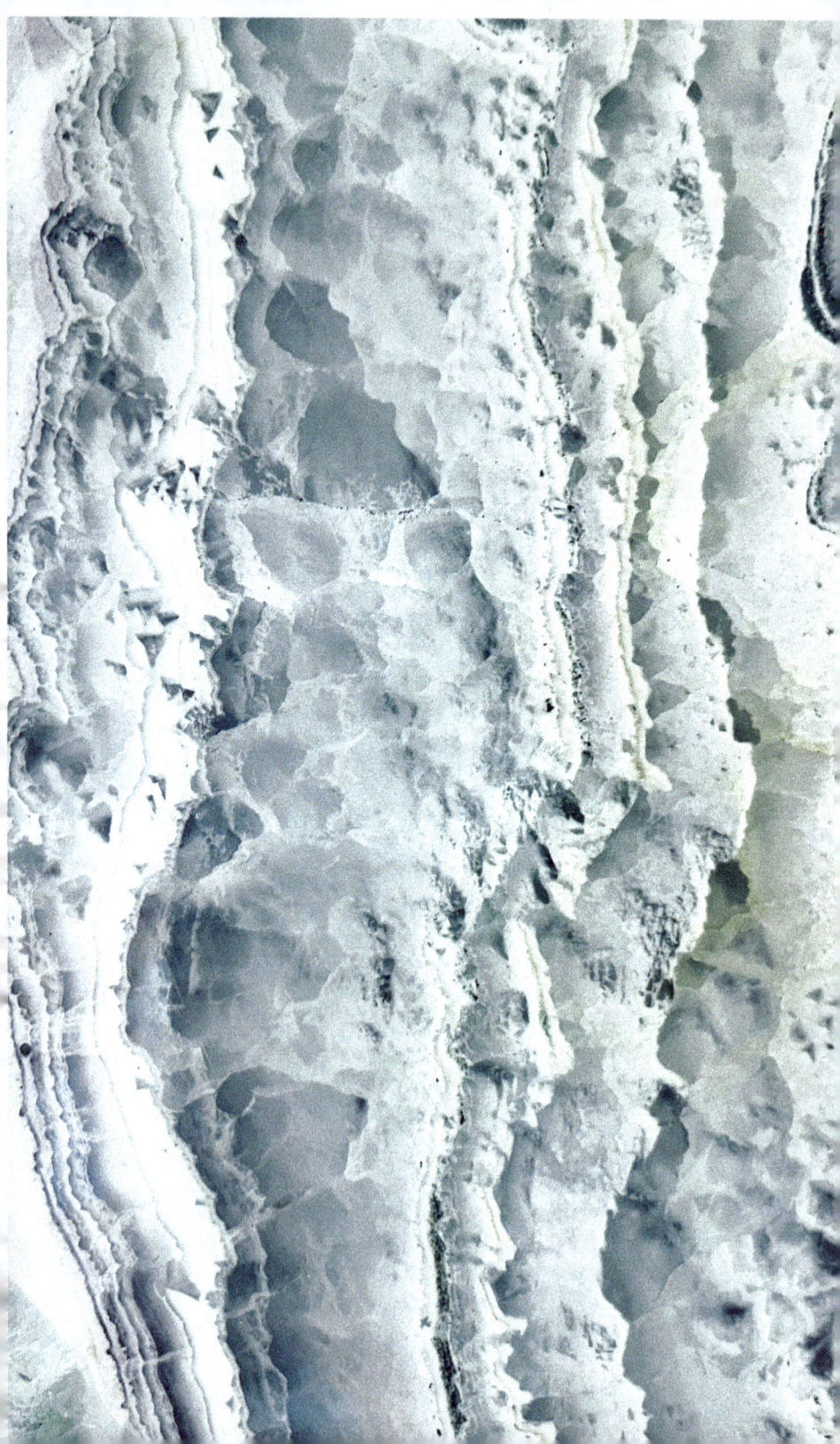

11- THREE VARIANTS OF LIFETHREAT

There are three fundamental variants of the lifethreat response.

Let's call the first one *pure shutdown*. Let's call the second one *tonic immobility*, which is also known as the freeze response. And the third one we will call *placate*. These responses have distinct autonomic neurology, and distinct biochemical signatures. Together they provide the three fundamental autonomic configurations undergirding chronic illness.

What I'd like to invite you to do in this chapter is to try to discern which of these patterns is active in your own situation. The first lifethreat response, *pure shutdown*, is characterized primarily by a high degree of collapse. It has very strong correlation with depression. At the level of the body, it is characterized by a feeling of physical collapse in the body, and the sense that the spine cannot hold itself up. The bounding box of the viscera collapses, and there is no muscle tone either in the pelvic floor or the respiratory diaphragm above it. The chest collapses. Stephen Porges, PhD calls this response *the dorsal vagal response*. In its most extreme formulation, you would simply pass out. It is characterized by strong inhibition on breathing, drop in heartrate, and a metabolic shut down. Its primary chemistry is endogenous opioids, which give us a subjective feeling of surreality, or a dream-like quality.

The second variant, *tonic immobility*, is a hybrid of the neurology of shutdown with high-level sympathetic tone. The combination of these two neurologies produces a state that has the primary quality of being rigid yet immobilized. The archetypal image here is of a deer in headlights. When people talk about being frozen in fear, for example, this is the archetype they're drawing from. In addition to the neurology, here incorporating the Movement System, the biochemistry is different. A pure shutdown state does not really have the presence of adrenaline and cortisol locked into it. This second presentation includes

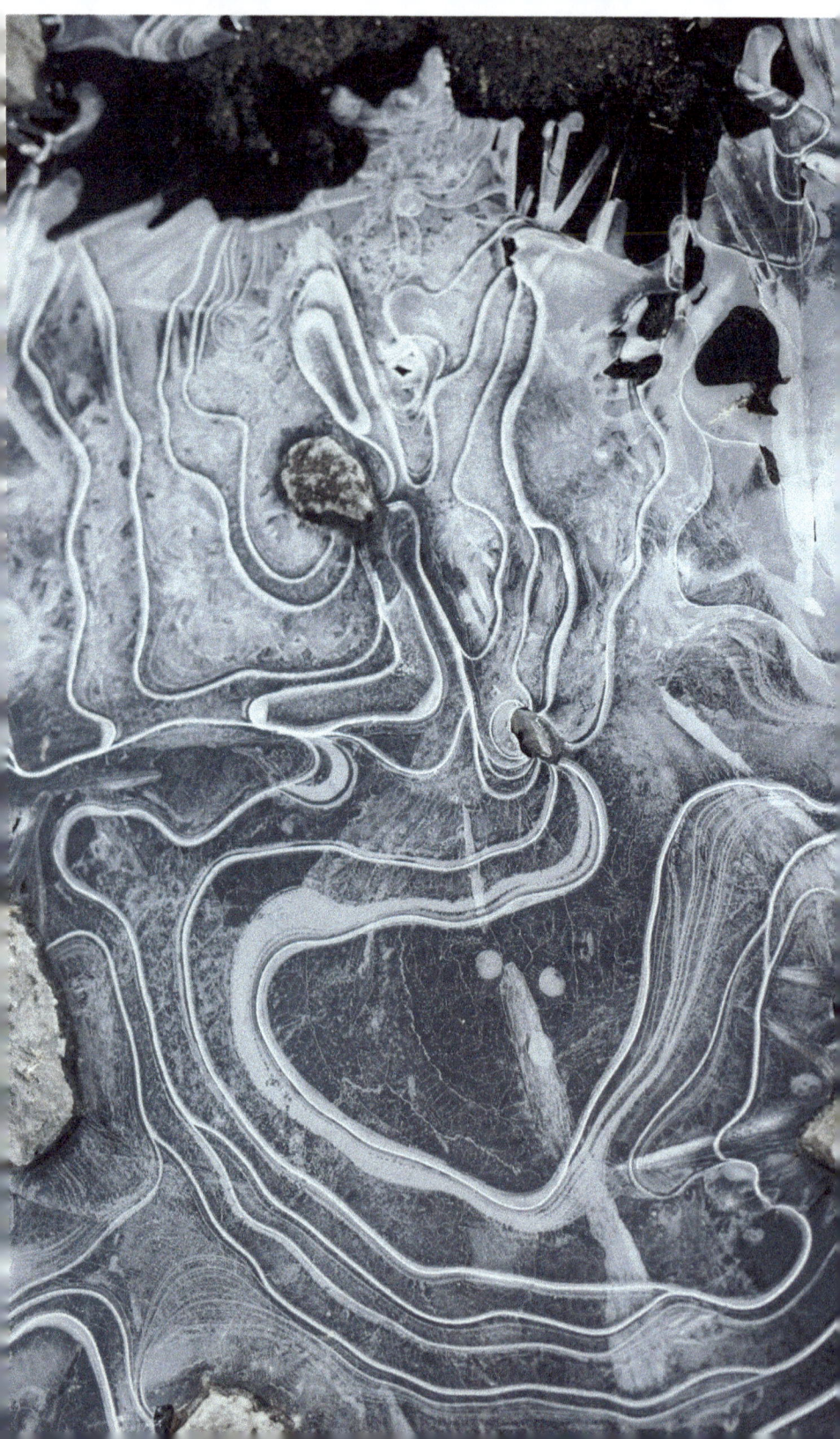

those two neuro-modulators. They tend to make the state feel very high arousal, yet immobilized. The sense is of the gears grinding, but being stuck.

Our third variant, *placate*, is a combination of the neurology of shutdown, with intent to experience greater safety by turning towards the threat. This combination is particularly prevalent in relational contact where a person is dealing with a violent Other. This kind of pattern can be learned early in life when we are contending with a parent who is violent, unpredictable, or mentally ill. It is a response that can be learned in dealing with someone who has addiction issues or is an alcoholic or flies into rages. Learned in dealing with someone who has a personality disorder, or is a narcissist, or a sociopath.

The paradox of this state is that it harnesses social neurobiology and social chemistry to attempt to deal with a lifethreat. This creates a biological paradox in the body, where we are attempting to open toward something that is causing us existential harm. In addition to the endogenous opioids of the shutdown state, placate can include oxytocin, which is the chemistry of love and bonding. In placate states, we bond to something that is trying to kill us.

The placate state is always pointed at someone or something else. It has an object outside of you.

Take a few minutes to reflect on the three variants of shutdown above. Take a minute to feel into your body, and to notice if any of these resonates with your own experience of yourself. Each of them is an adaptive response to lifethreat. Please realize also that each of these states exists on a continuum of intensity. There is a full-blown version of the state, and a micro version of the state. A full-blown pure shutdown response might involve passing out, while a micro version might be not remembering where we put our wallet.

Each of these states probably kept you alive through experiences that otherwise would have been unendurable. Each of them also extracts a profound metabolic cost from us, particularly if it becomes chronic and non-resolving. Getting clear about which of these primary patterns undergirds your own experience of chronic illness will help you begin to unwind it. Each of these is, ultimately, an autonomic *habit*. Each of us has a repertoire of responses available to us for responding to different kinds of threat. As we have discussed earlier in the book, many of these habits were set for us very early in life as adaptive responses to our family situations, which we could not control as small children. As adults, however, we have much greater optionality. We can learn new ways of managing stress and threat. We can unlearn coping mechanisms and autonomic habits that no longer serve us. We can help bring back responses that are not currently on our autonomic menus.

I realize in writing this that some of you reading it will feel like this is not possible. To those of you I would like you to know that we have helped people in their 60s and 70s relearn these kinds of autonomic habits. We have worked with people suffering from complex chronic illness, Complex Regional Pain Syndrome, Parkinson's disease, Lupus, and other chronic conditions. By developing autonomic awareness, learning autonomic fluency, and gaining new skills around how you respond to distress, and welcome trustworthy connection, it is possible to help your body reset some of the foundation baselines for how you process experiences. Although this is not the only thing required to heal from complex chronic illness, if you do not address this aspect of the disease, you are failing to address the underlying energy processing templates that gave rise to it in the first place.

In the next section of the book, we will explore some of the foundation frameworks required to become more aware of what is happening autonomically in your body and mind.

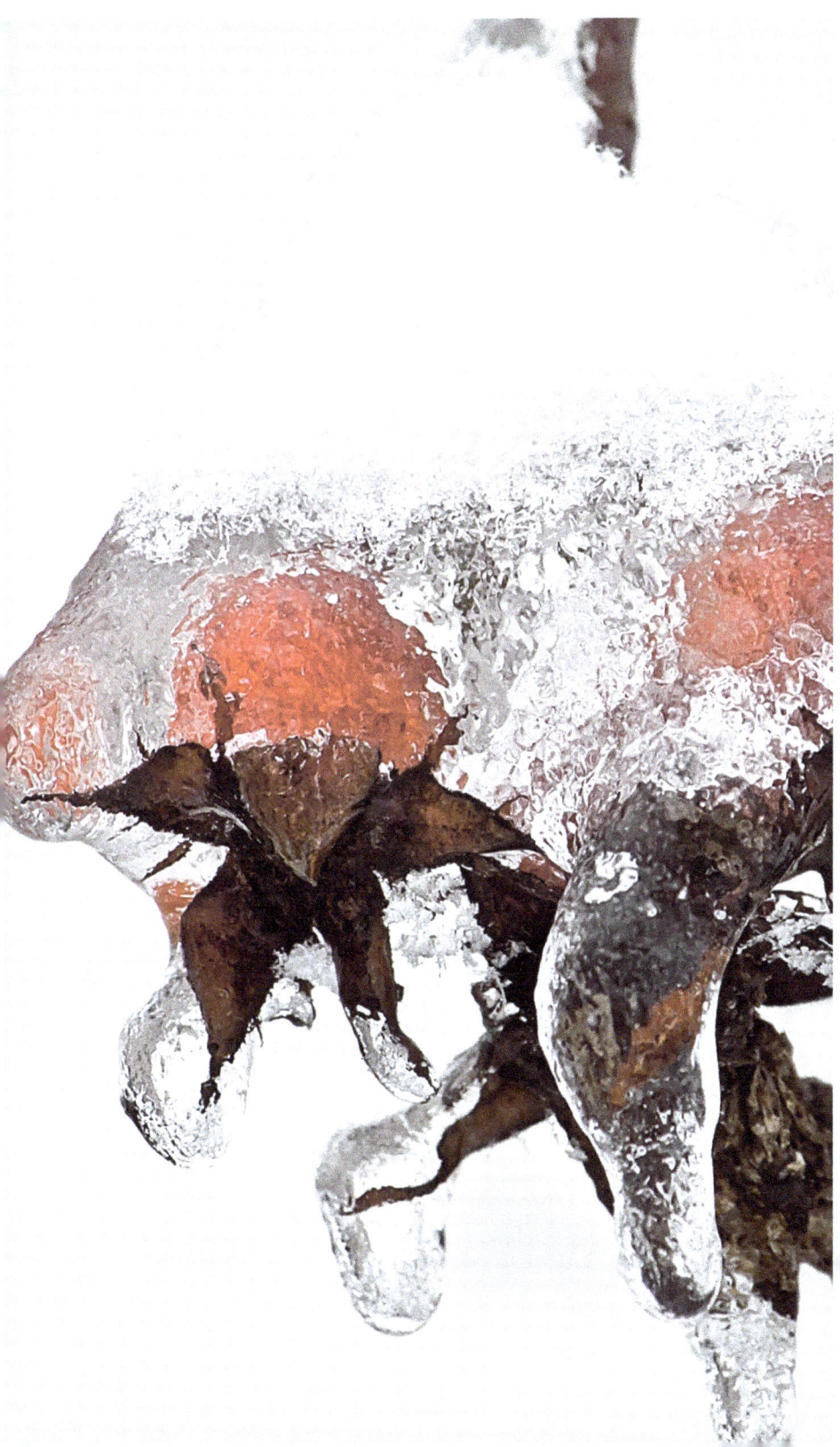

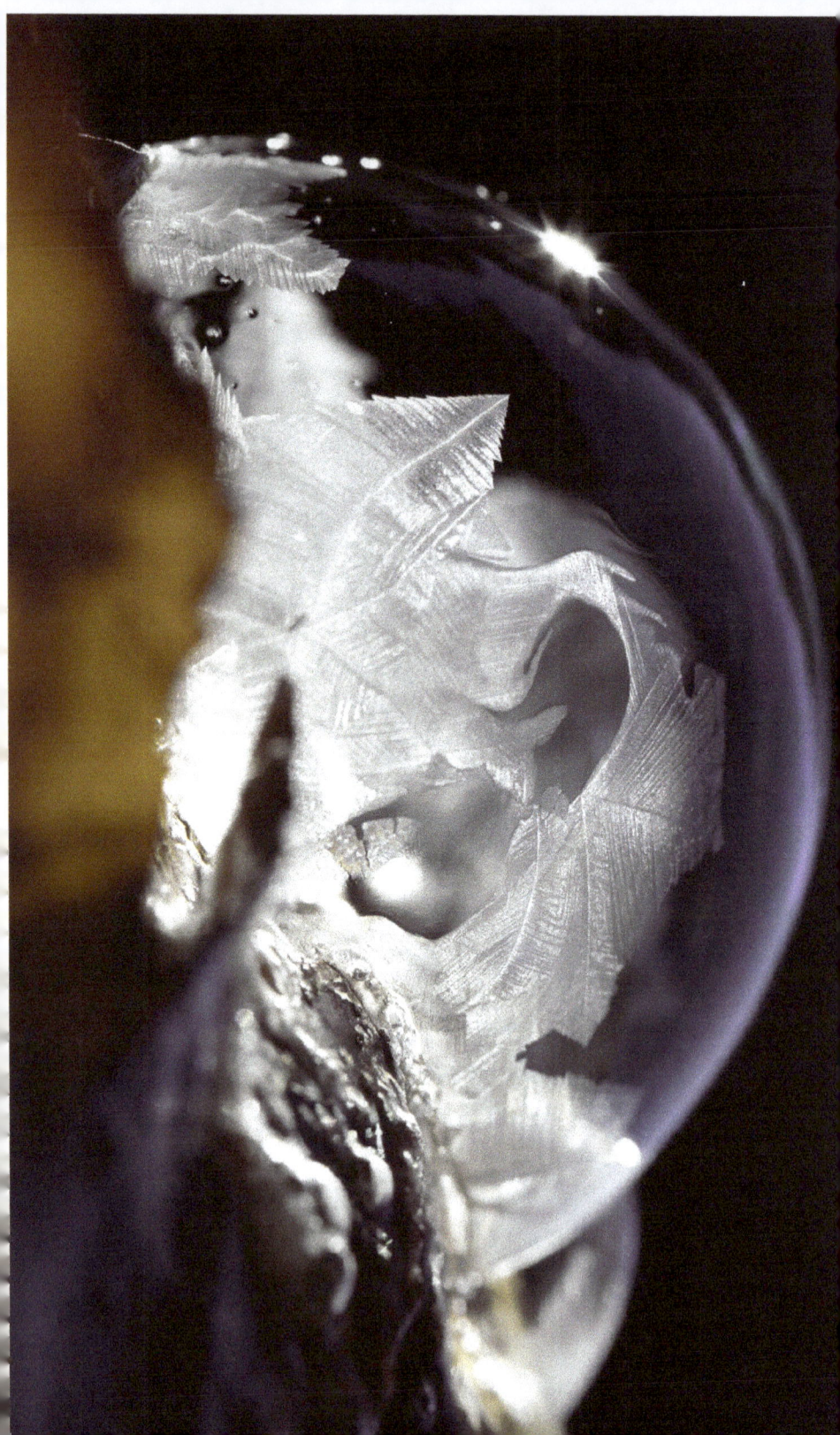

PART TWO: FRAMEWORKS

12- SELF AS WATER

Think of yourself as a water droplet. Water can exist in three phases. Liquid, solid, or gas. It transitions between these phases based on energy in the form of temperature. This flexibility of form permits it to continue to exist across an extraordinary range of temperature.

Your Autonomic Nervous System is just like this. Based on its present-moment assessment of safety, danger, or lifethreat, it shifts between different states. The body that you are wearing now, the body that you are living in, is a historical recording of your life history autonomically.

In this analogy, the more of the water droplet of you that exists in a liquid water state, the healthier you are. The more of the water droplet that exists as steam, the more it means that you are carrying around unresolved allostatic load in the form of unmetabolized fight-or-flight responses. The more of the water droplet that exists as ice, the more it means that you are carrying around unresolved allostatic load in the form of unmetabolized shutdown responses.

If you are contending with chronic illness, we already know that a critical percentage of your water droplet is in the form of ice.

The water analogy is important for a further reason, which is that when we think about autonomic healing, it is crucial that we are able to discern whether the allostatic loads that the body is holding onto, that it has been unable to metabolize and clear, are in the form of archived fight-flight responses, or archived shutdown responses. To say this another way, we need to know whether what is not liquid water is steam or ice. This discernment will determine how we intervene. If we do not make this distinction, we will apply modes of intervention that are at best irrelevant, and at worse harmful. If you are trying to get steam back to liquid water, you cool it. But you can cool ice all day long, and nothing will happen. Many of the standard interventions for stress do not apply to shutdown states, or are contra-indicated.

My firm has done extensive research, for example, on types of meditation that are contra-indicated when someone is in a shutdown state. Most meditative practices you would encounter in most meditation lineages are directly contra-indicated if you are in a shutdown state. They will in fact further increase dissociation, driving you deeper into shutdown, not bringing you out of it. The failure of the mindfulness movement to recognize this is a result of its broad lack of understanding of autonomic physiology. In order to have skillful means working with autonomic states, we have to have clarity about their composition.

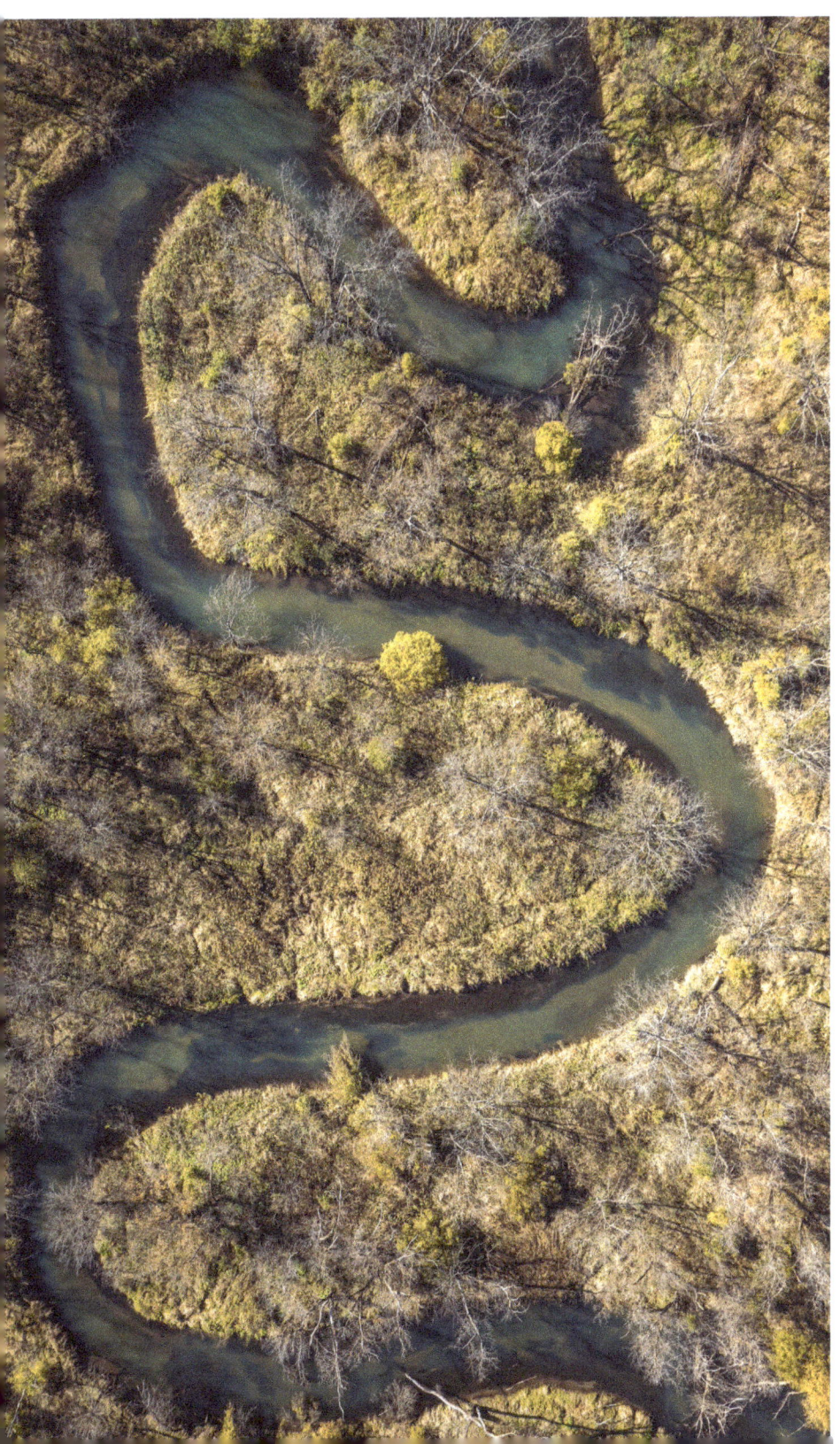

13- MINDBODY SYSTEM

The Autonomic Nervous System is the neural architecture of the mindbody connection. For this reason, stress-related disease is always mindbody. It will always have physical components, because the purview of the ANS is the regulation of your internal milieu, and it will always have psychological components, because this regulation governs how you feel.

This means that stress-related issues are inherently problematic for allopathic medicine, which is organized around an artificial partitioning of the mind from the body. Allopathic medicine does not have either a conceptual schema or a practitioner classification system that is capable of clearly perceiving the entire range of autonomic phenomena altered by stress-related disorders holistically. For this reason, most people with complex chronic illness have had the exhausting and endlessly frustrating experience of being shuffled around through allopathic medical systems, from General Practitioners to various specialists and back. You see the GP with digestive issues, and are then referred to gastro-enterology. The interventions of the gastro-enterologist impact upon your mood and you are referred to psychiatry. The side effects of psych meds create further physical symptoms, or make you less alert, and you are referred elsewhere. And on and on and on. At no point in this referral chain is allopathic medicine capable of stepping back and recognizing that it is dealing with systematic deflections of a single autonomic system. If you tell the gastro-enterologist about emotional symptoms they look at you funny. If you tell the psychiatrist about inflammation they look at you funny. Allopathic medicine is fundamentally structurally inequipped to effectively treat stress-related disorders.

This is actually a huge problem for them, because 60-80% of what brings people into primary care is stress-related. It means allopathic medicine is not able to effectively treat most of what is wrong with modern people.

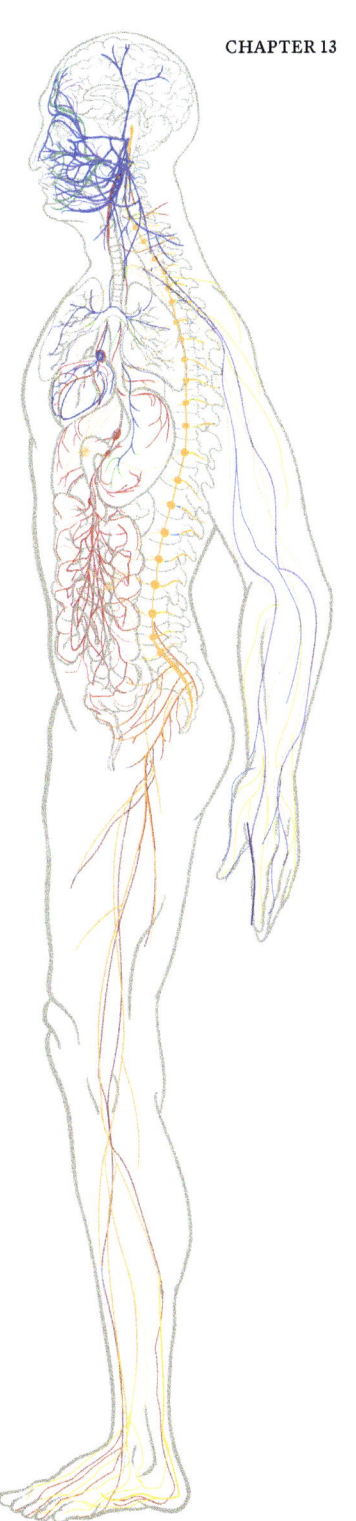

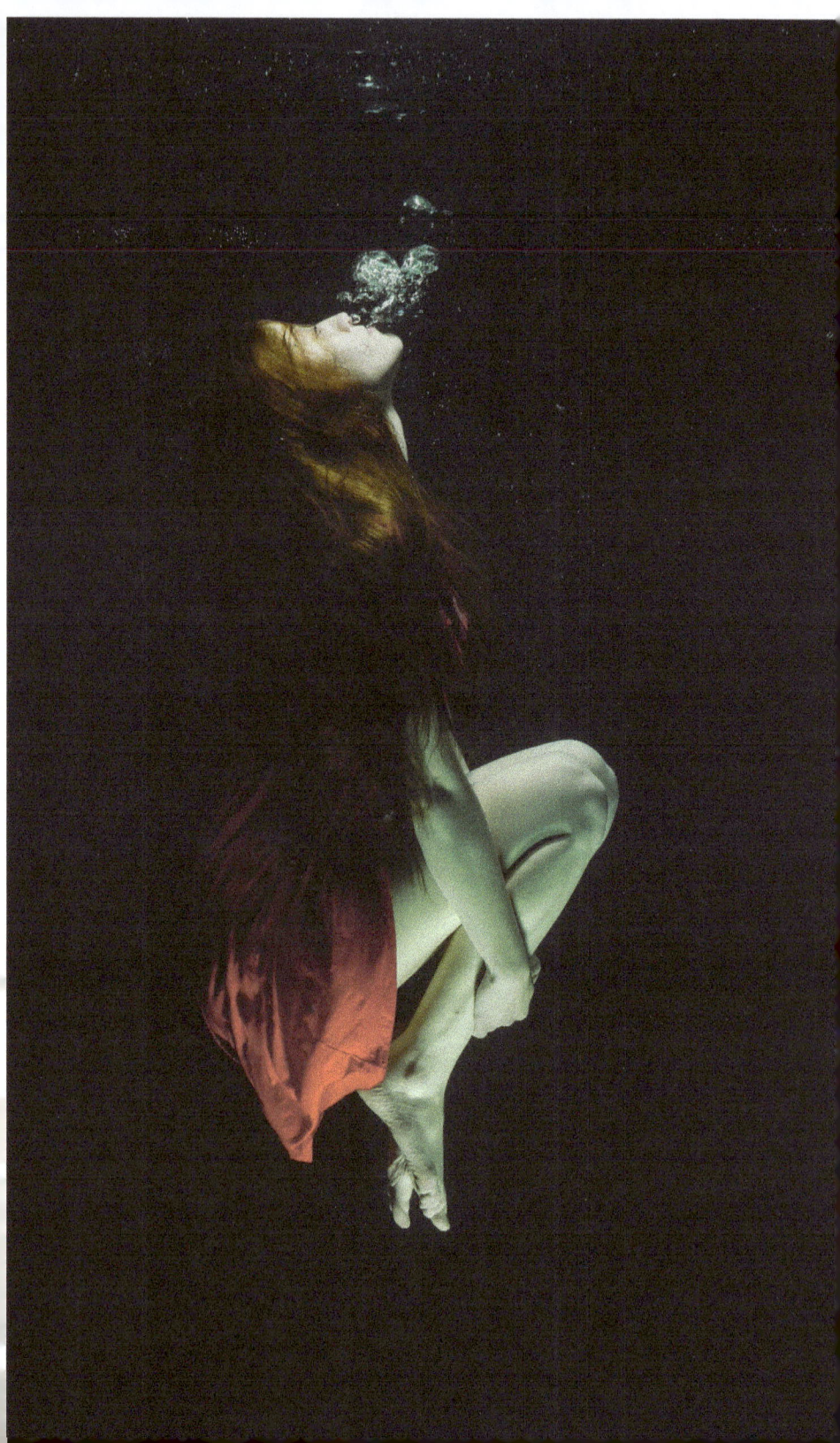

14- IT'S NOT IN YOUR HEAD

Furthermore, when we are dealing with complex chronic illness, we are often encouraged to seek mental health support in the form of therapy. While I'm a huge fan of therapy, self-reflection, and the development of awareness generally, it is important to recognize that talk therapy does not actually touch the places in the deep nervous system that are governing the templates through which you process experience. It is also not equipped to help you move through the process of outflowing accumulated allostatic loads.

Furthermore, the solidification of the stories that we have about events, histories, things we have experienced, and things we have witnessed can get in the way of us actually addressing the felt visceral embodied componentry of what happened. The relationship between language and experience is very potent. Stories can be a way of containing energies that we do not want to feel. In order to get to the visceral and felt layers at which experience is actually held in the body, sometimes we have to get underneath or beyond the stories we have about what happened.

I'm not denigrating our sense-making abilities: I'm just noting that stories are a double-edged sword. Therapies that include the body, and are awareness-based, are the most likely to be able to work with the complexity of mindbody issues present in chronic illness: to get to the depths where experience is processed physiologically in the body.

I have personally been impressed by the body-centered (or somatic) therapies in this regard, of which there are many. These approaches tend to be holistic, acknowledge the depth of the mindbody connection, and tilt toward the experiential, utilizing movement, touch, and other direct experiences during therapy. Most help us build awareness of bodily sensations. These modalities include Hakomi Method, Sensori-Motor Psychotherapy, and certain lineages of Somatic Experiencing®. If you are in the US, the United States Association for Body Psychotherapy (http://www.usabp.org) hosts a practitioner directory that can help you find a somatic therapist in your area. Somatic therapy is ideally done with someone face-to-face. Although often practitioners will offer to do it remotely, you'll be happier with the results of being in-person with a practitioner.

15- ECOLOGICAL MODEL

One of the most frustrating things about complex chronic illness is that the healing process is not linear. Whereas a broken bone mends itself directly, heals in a way that makes steady progress, the healing of chronic illness is rarely linear. You get better, you get worse, you get better again, you get much worse. You get much better.

This can prove deeply disheartening, particularly if we do not understand it. The dance between feeling worse, and our psychological state– feelings of powerlessness or hopelessness– puts people onto a seesaw, watching themselves rise and fall seemingly at the whim of something that they do not understand, the pivot that raises and lowers them out of reach, and this can develop a sense of learned helplessness where it doesn't seem that we have any sense of agency in our own healing.

Furthermore, because chronic illness is the result of the complex interaction between neurological, immune, and endocrine systems, it is often difficult to discern what is making us feel worse when symptoms flair, because there can be time delays between cause and effect. Again, the net impact of this disconnect between call-and-response is disheartening, and can make us feel disempowered, which furthers the cycle of shutdown.

I would like to introduce here an ecological model to help you have a deeper felt sense of both the process of how complex chronic illness develops, and what we are doing when we heal it.

When I was young, I spent a good deal of time on the Meramec River in Missouri, where my family had a cabin. Usually we started visiting in late April or May, after the heavy rains of winter. One of the first things I always did on arriving was to go down to the water to look at the sandbars, because every year they moved. Each year the heavy winter rains rushed

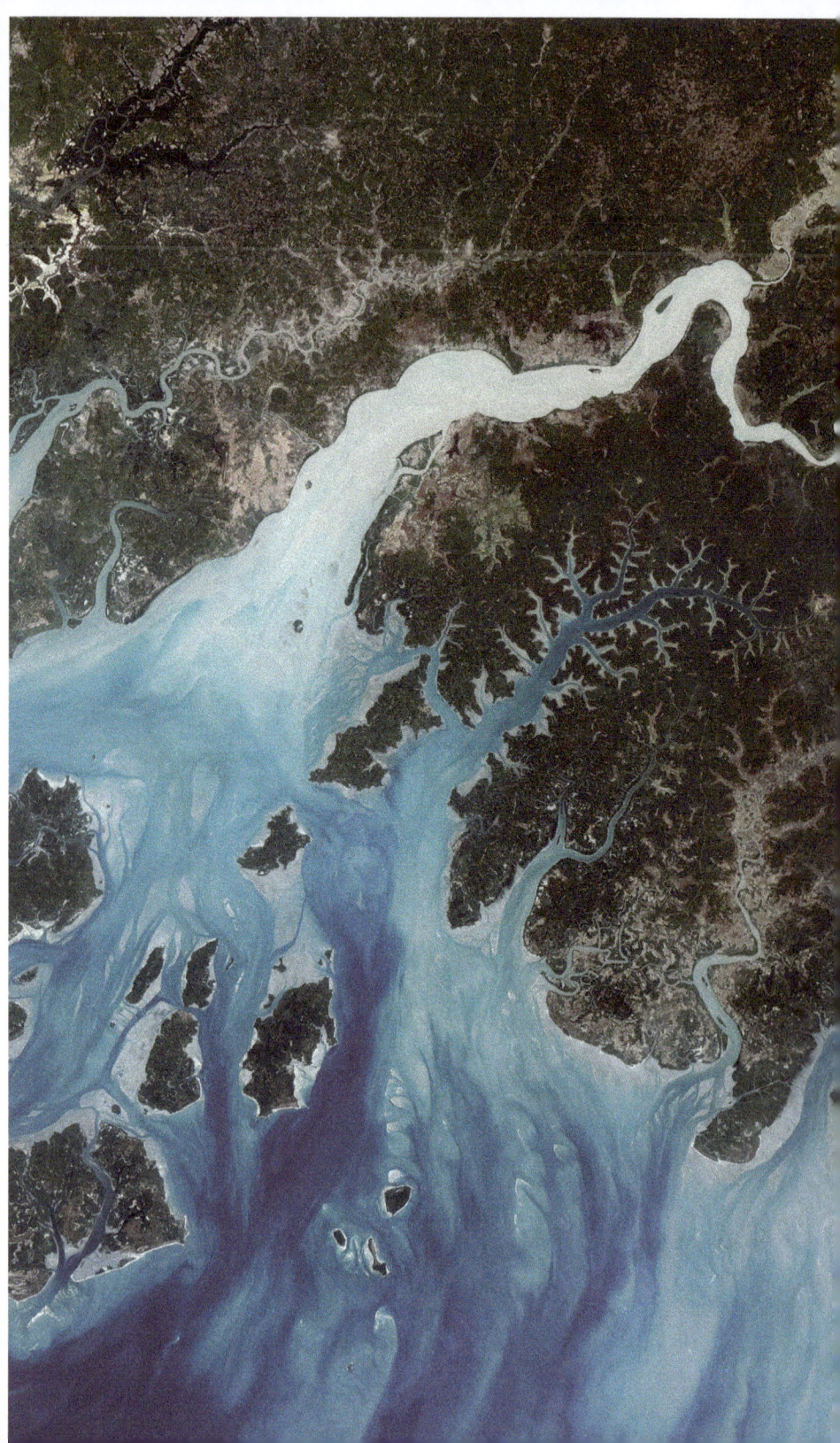

through the river channel, and the volume of water, and what it was carrying, interacted with the river bed, pushing the silt and sand around.

I find it helpful to think about your life experiences as the water rushing through the channel that push your physiological baseline from year to year. Early adverse life experiences, and the energy-processing templates that we engage to deal with them, specifically *pure shutdown*, *tonic immobility*, and *placating*, exhibit shaping force on the way that the river of experience flows across our bodies.

Over time these autonomic habits begin to move the setpoints in our physiology the same way that the winter rains move the sandbars.

Certain kinds of interventions may be akin to damming the river: pharmaceutical interventions are sometimes like this. But if you want to really recover your health, the process that we are engaged in is one of changing the way that experience flows through your system so that the sandbars move back in the opposite direction.

When we look carefully at the etiology of chronic illness, we have to grapple with the reality that it usually develops over decades.[1] Although its onset can seem sudden, we don't typically develop symptoms until there have been fundamental changes in the riverbed.

The long game of transforming chronic illness is to use the same elemental forces that shifted the setpoints of our physiology out of balance to bring them back into balance.

I hope that this chapter helps you to change the view of what chronic illness is, your sense of patience in dealing with it, and

---

1 Sometimes there is a pre-existing autonomic baseline from early adversity that gets pushed across a threshold by an illness (COVID-19, some other virus) or a particular life stressor.

your understanding of the timescales required.

I am not in any way here dismissing the role of radical intervention, or pharmaceuticals at all. I'm simply hoping to reframe the way you think about the process of transformation: to move it out of the too-simple ways people often think about it into a more ecological model of altering physiological baselines.

16- RELATING

The primary concept that I want to land for you in this book– its central teaching– is that how we feel in our bodies and minds is *a result of how we relate*.

The Autonomic Nervous System is the neural architecture of the mindbody connection, and it shapes the energy-processing templates that govern our experience. But the primary content flowing through these energy-processing templates is our *relating*.

At the deepest level, the nervous system is all about relating. It is a system that translates between exteriors and interiors, constantly taking the temperature of our interactions, and modulating the body's processes in response.

Most people do not think about the nervous system through this lens of the deep strata of our relating. We fail to recognize the way it is mediating between us and other people. In our focus on its sensory and motor components we have lost sight of the reality that much of what governs how our nervous systems work is driven by what is required to relate to the people around us.

My mentor Stephen Porges, PhD, Developer of the Polyvagal Theory, and one of the world's leading experts on the relationship between the Autonomic Nervous System and behavior points out that human wellbeing is social in nature. Most of us deeply fail to understand the degree to which, as social mammals, our wellbeing is socially constructed. The corollary to what Porges is saying, which becomes apparent in the case of chronic illness, is that *illbeing* is also social in nature. Or, said slightly differently, illbeing is the byproduct of interacting socially with others who make us feel habitually unsafe.

The reason that most modern people spend so much time living in their heads– residing in their thinking– is that it feels shitty to most people to live in their bodies.

And the reason it feels shitty is because most modern people feel chronically unsafe. This lack of a felt sense of safety has many flavors, yet there are only so many physiological ways that the Autonomic Nervous System can respond to it, because there are only so many combinations of neuroception, autonomic neurology, and neurochemistry.

Unsafety can take the form of chronicity of the flight response, which is the root driver of anxiety. It can take the form of chronicity of the fight response, which is the root driver of combativeness. It can take the form of appeasing, where sociality is overlaid on top of a fight-fight response, and we turn toward a source of social threat to disarm it. We begin to identify with the states that we spend the most time in, be they health-creating (*salutogenic*) or disease-creating (*pathogenic*). If my experience of unsafety pushes me into habitual flight responses, I start to understand myself as an anxious person.

If you are reading this book because you have chronic illness, what is more likely is that your own chronic experience of unsafety took a different neurological route, which involved the shutdown response in some way.

17- AUTONOMIC SELF

I imagine us having an autonomic self, different from our ordinary egoic sense of self, that is the autonomic intelligence that governs how we respond to safety, danger, and lifethreat. This autonomic self learns from our experiences which defensive responses are most adaptive. Its baseline objective is to keep us alive. As long as we survive, it is doing its job.

In the house I grew up in, although my father was not a violent person, he was not skillful with anger. He was a young man when I was born, and I learned pretty early in life that if I responded to feeling unsafe by getting angry with him, he would get *more* angry with me. At the time my body learned this lesson deeply I probably weighed less than fifty pounds, and he probably weighed about a hundred and fifty pounds. At that point in my life, if things had gotten physical, I would have lost a fight every single time.

Because I'm not stupid, anger eventually came off of my menu as a viable autonomic response. This was not a conscious decision that my ordinary sense of self made: rather it was an autonomic evaluation. Like an autonomic tributary that simply dries up because a barrier is erected across its enterance, my body noticed that if I responded to feeling threatened by getting angry with my father, the result of this was much more frightening. So I stopped doing this. *Do I want to have a person three times my size screaming at me?* I do not. I guess I won't do that.

With the fight response off the menu, and based on my early experience of displacement at seven years old, I moved into a more chronic shutdown response. I spent most of my adolescence living in this state, disconnected from my body, and living largely in my thinking, which is the place that most people go when it either doesn't feel good to live in our bodies, or we simply cannot feel them anymore.

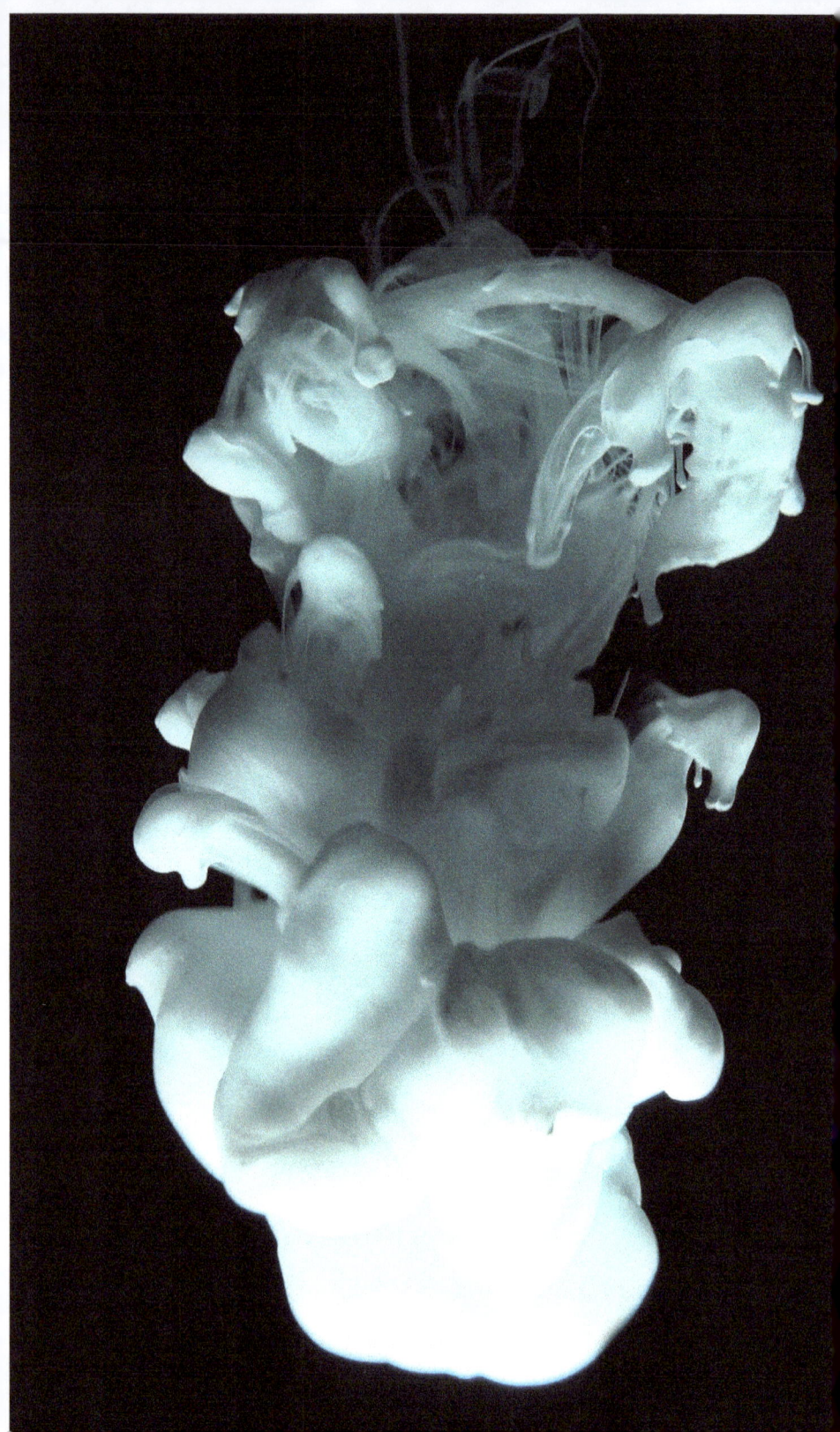

Because I was pretty shut down, because the flow of vitality through my body was quite restricted, there was a limit on the amount of emotion that I could tolerate flowing through my body.

I don't think it is an accident that I learned to meditate. If your vitality is constricted, meditating is a way to begin to contact your interior in a manner that is very controlled. In addition, because I was already very shut down, I could tolerate sitting still for long periods of time, since I was already immobilized.

I credit meditation, and bodyscanning practices in particular, with my learning how to make visceral contact with my interior once again; with learning how to feel myself on the inside. But like many people drawn to meditation, part of the reason that it felt good was because I was already really shut down. Having a controlled context in which to feel myself inwardly was necessary for me, both because my body had restricted the flow-through of vitality so dramatically, and because if energy and emotion started moving through my system, I would feel really out-of-control. For a very long time I confused dissociation with equanimity.

I thought that I was a balanced chill meditative dude. In reality, I was shutdown and dissociated. The difference is important. Equanimity means that you are able to hold the mast of the boat upright on stormy seas. It means that in the tumult of waves of emotion and energy rising and falling you have learned to keep steady. Dissociation means that your bodymind system cannot permit energy and emotion to flow through it. Put another way, if the sea is frozen, you aren't really dealing with stormy seas because there are not waves in ice.

So meditation became a way for me to initiate contact with myself, a way to experience enough visceral safety in a controlled environment that I could begin to feel myself from inside, begin to occupy myself again. Yet I still could not process emotion and energy moving through my body in realtime. As I began to have more visceral contact with my body, to feel myself inwardly once again, I would still accumulate feeling, and then I would still have to sit, sometimes for hours, in order to metabolize it.

Part of what I began to discern, as I began to build a baseline understanding of autonomic physiology in my thirties, was the way that I had constricted certain energy processing templates (specifically the fight response) early in life. Because my body could not go here, could not fight back, could not respond with anger, I was simply moving into shutdown and accumulating that allostatic load. And this same pattern was happening all across my life.

I had become the prisoner of a set of habits of autonomic relating, because I didn't have a full menu of autonomic options for responding to threat.

As an adult, decades later, there was then a distinct phase of my own trauma healing process where I had to re-learn to allow myself to get angry. I had to bring this physiological response back onto my biological menu.

I want to notice both the intelligence of this autonomic self, and its responses, and the ways that ultimately they proved limiting. I want to notice that sometimes we have to unlearn habitual ways of relating, and go back to open up old pathways that fell off of our menus, sometimes decades ago, because it was too dangerous for us to deploy them at the time.

18- BODY AS COMPASS

If we start from the opposite premise allopathic medicine has adopted, from a premise that begins with unity, and we view the bodymind as a continuum that is fundamentally neurologically integrated (*which it is*) we can take the deeply radical step of treating our symptoms as meaningful.

I had a conversation once with a woman who developed a lineage of somatic movement therapy who told me, *Cancer is a verb*. This assertion really stayed with me, because what she was saying is that a disease is not a *thing*. It is not a noun. It is a process.

We are taught to think about dysfunction mechanistically. But imbalance is a process that unfolds. And the place that we can have some agency in engaging with this process is at the level of the felt, and this engagement becomes much more useful if we are able to regard symptoms as a manifestation of intelligence.

If you get headaches, the fact that they are in your head is meaningful. If you feel like you are going to throw up, the fact that you feel like you are going to throw up is meaningful. Our bodies have this extraordinary ability to show us where energy and experience is getting stuck.

Most of the ancient holistic medical systems of the world, from Ayurveda to Traditional Chinese Medicine, deeply embrace this awareness: it is how they diagnose. Beginning with a view that the body is fundamentally intelligent, that part of its job is to metabolize our experiences, it views the location, texture, and experience of symptoms as being meaningful.

Many of us have been trained by modernity to want to make pain disappear. If you have a headache you take Tylenol, you don't ask yourself why you have a headache and not a stomach ache. But I would like to encourage you, if you are really interested in healing, to take a very sober look at this reaction. Allopathic medicine has a tendency to say something like this: *If you do not like the reading on the compass, smash the compass.*

In my personal and clinical experience, most of the time this is a terrible idea. Instead, what I would suggest, is, *If you do not like the reading on the compass, get very curious about why your compass is pointing in that direction.*

Let us make the radical assertion that instead of some professional, instead of a physician, or a psychotherapist, or another trained specialist, you are actually the person most likely to understand what is happening inside you. I realize that this is almost frightening to many people, but consider. You are the only person who has been inside your experience from the beginning. You are the only one who has been there in all of the moments of your life. Even the most experienced professional in the world is only hearing second-hand about what you have lived.

The living edge of your healing process emerges at the moment you turn toward your symptoms with curiosity and ask– *Why is the pain showing up in this particular way?*

PART THREE: APPLICATION

19- PRACTICING SOMETHING NEW

What I am specifically *not* going to talk about in this practice and application section of the book are things related to infection, and/or immune and endocrine conditions, despite their obvious relevance, because these things are outside of my purview. While all of these are deep and consistent features of chronic illness, what I will try to do in this section is keep the focus specifically on the autonomic components of this process.

I don't want you to think of this book as a standalone treatment armamentarium. Rather, what I'd like to do here is continue to help you get a handle on places where you can become more agentic about giving yourself more beneficial autonomic inputs to support your well-being, with awareness that this is just a piece of the total puzzle of your healing work.

There are three broad categories of autonomic neurological intervention that I would like to think about with you.

METABOLIZING ALLOSTATIC LOADS

The first of these is the continued physiological metabolizing of trauma. As we have been discussing throughout the text, a lot of the autonomic habits that undergird chronic illness are learned early in childhood. So, one of the core practices that will continue to engage is looking to actually physiologically transform and outflow these allostatic loads.

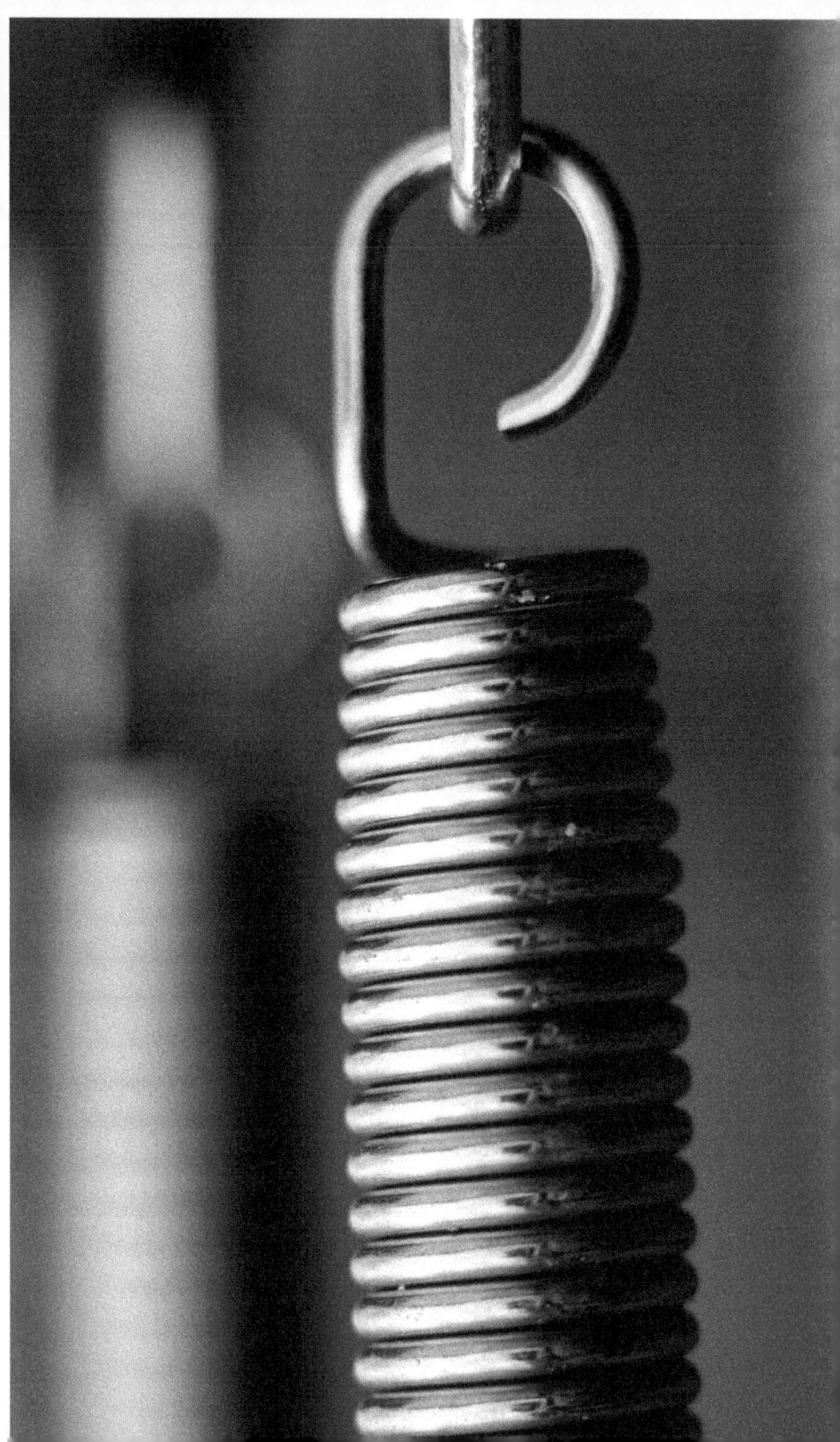

GETTING ALTERNATIVE STRESS RESPONSES ON THE MENU

The second category of practice/process is what I would call *getting alternative stress responses on the menu*. This has to do with helping your deep nervous system have more options for how it responds to stress and threat, such that it does not default into a variant of shutdown response.

EVOKING CONNECTION STATES

And then the third category of response is to continue to augment and evoke connection states. This category has to do with increasing the health-creating inputs to our deep nervous system. I have written extensively about this in *The Neurobiology of Connection: Re-Wilding Your Deep Nervous System for Wellbeing*. With some specific alterations that are particular to working with complex chronic illness, this final section of the text will therefore focus on practices that address these three categories of transforming our autonomic baselines.

20- METABOLIZING ALLOSTATIC LOADS

Something I hear fairly often from people who have histories of early childhood adversity that resulted in their systems moving preferentially into shutdown responses is, "But I don't *feel* stressed out."

I think there are probably a few reasons people say this. One of them is that when most people think about stress, they are thinking about fight-or-flight responses. When people say they don't feel stressed out, they're being sincere. They don't feel highly aroused, irritated, agitated, anxious, or fearful. They don't feel tense. They do not have adrenaline coursing through their systems. Yet although mainstream medicine doesn't talk about it, although most people have no conceptualization of it, there are different types of allostatic loads. What most people think about as stress includes adrenaline and cortisol and jitters and teeth-clenching and muscle tension: what we might call *hot* stress. But most shutdown responses do not include either of these chemistries or any of these somatic attributes. Just because you do not feel stressed out, does not mean that the body is not archiving tremendous reservoirs of stress. The stress is simply of a different kind and quality. It is *cold* stress.

By the time it becomes chronic illness, most of these reservoirs are locked into metabolic and physiological changes in bodily systems. Disruption of digestion is the indirect evidence of accumulated stress. Constriction of breath is the indirect evidence of accumulated stress. Chronic illness is the cumulative indirect evidence of accumulated stress. So a more useful question to ask is, *How might stress be archived in my body that I am not aware of?*

Because of the specific nature of shutdown responses, and the fact that one of the things they do is decrease interoceptive awareness, people who have a history of shutdown responses also often don't necessarily *feel* very much. So if shutdown is one of our go-to responses, there is probably a lot of stuff happening in our bodies that we have learned NOT to feel. Going into shutdown shifts the neurobiological setpoints in our inward sensitivity to the felt. Shutdown responses are in fact dissociative. So where there is accumulation of unmetabolized shutdown response there are typically interoceptive deficits.

Because of the invisibility of these kinds of stress to most of us who are embodying them, the fact that they simply take parts (or all) of the body offline at a feeling level, the work of metabolizing these kinds of loads is often best undertaken with the help of someone else. It is hard to see what we cannot see; it is hard to feel what we cannot feel; it is hard to notice what we are not aware of.

Having someone who is a skilled autonomic practitioner who can help reflect back to us the places where we are shut down, where our voice loses affect, where we disconnect from the ground, where we disconnect from our bodies, where we armor up against feeling– someone to help skillfully disrupt the numerous ways that we have learned not to know what the body knows: this is helpful if not downright necessary.

Furthermore, the metabolizing of allostatic loads is not a generic process. It is quite individual. The overwhelming experiences that caused you to accumulate the loads in the first place are archived in your body. Addressing them means creating a context where they can be worked with directly, and this is the particular province of trauma healing. While we can discuss the principles of it in a book, the physiological experience of this is what you need, and it cannot take the form of simply awareness-building or exercises.

Overwhelming experiences are particular. They involve specific situations, and specific autonomic responses, specific movements of the body. The refined somatic trauma healing lineages work with this specificity.

In the car accident, the vehicle begins to spin in a particular direction, which causes our body to shift in the seat in a particular way, tensioning a particular set of muscles, and impacts our vestibular system with the application of particular vectors of force. The impact happens at a specific angle. The racing of the heart on inhaling the smell of crushed metal happens at a particular moment, and when we jump out of the car, the primary lift is from one leg, not the other.

Unwinding the accident somatically, at the level of the body, requires attending to the specifics of these sensations, and that is not something that can be done generically through a set of exercises.

You need to do that kind of process with someone skilled in tracking autonomically.

While the overwhelming experience I am describing, of a car accident, is a category of overwhelming experience, and could be referred to as being a type of *shock* trauma, often the antecedents to chronic illness are relational traumas, which are classified as *developmental* traumas.

While Somatic Experiencing® is a modality that works very effectively with shock trauma, developmental trauma is outside of its scope. The modality needs to be well indicated for the form of injury. In the appendix to this book is a list of different lineages of somatically-oriented trauma therapies with enough alignment to the Autonomics framework that they will not contradict things you are learning here, with a brief explanation of their relative scope of practice. This is the experiential work indicated by an understanding of the autonomic foundation of chronic illness.

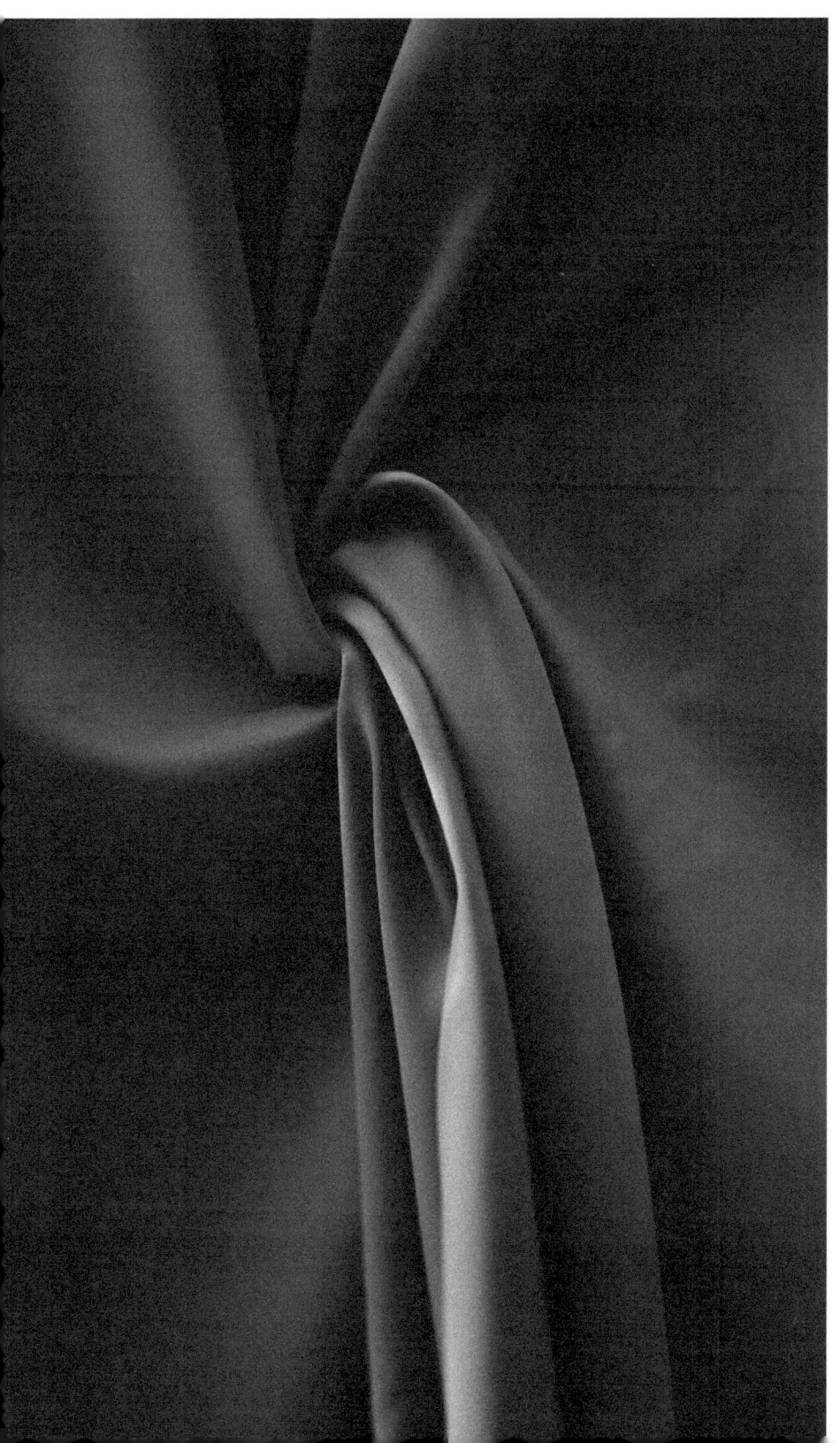

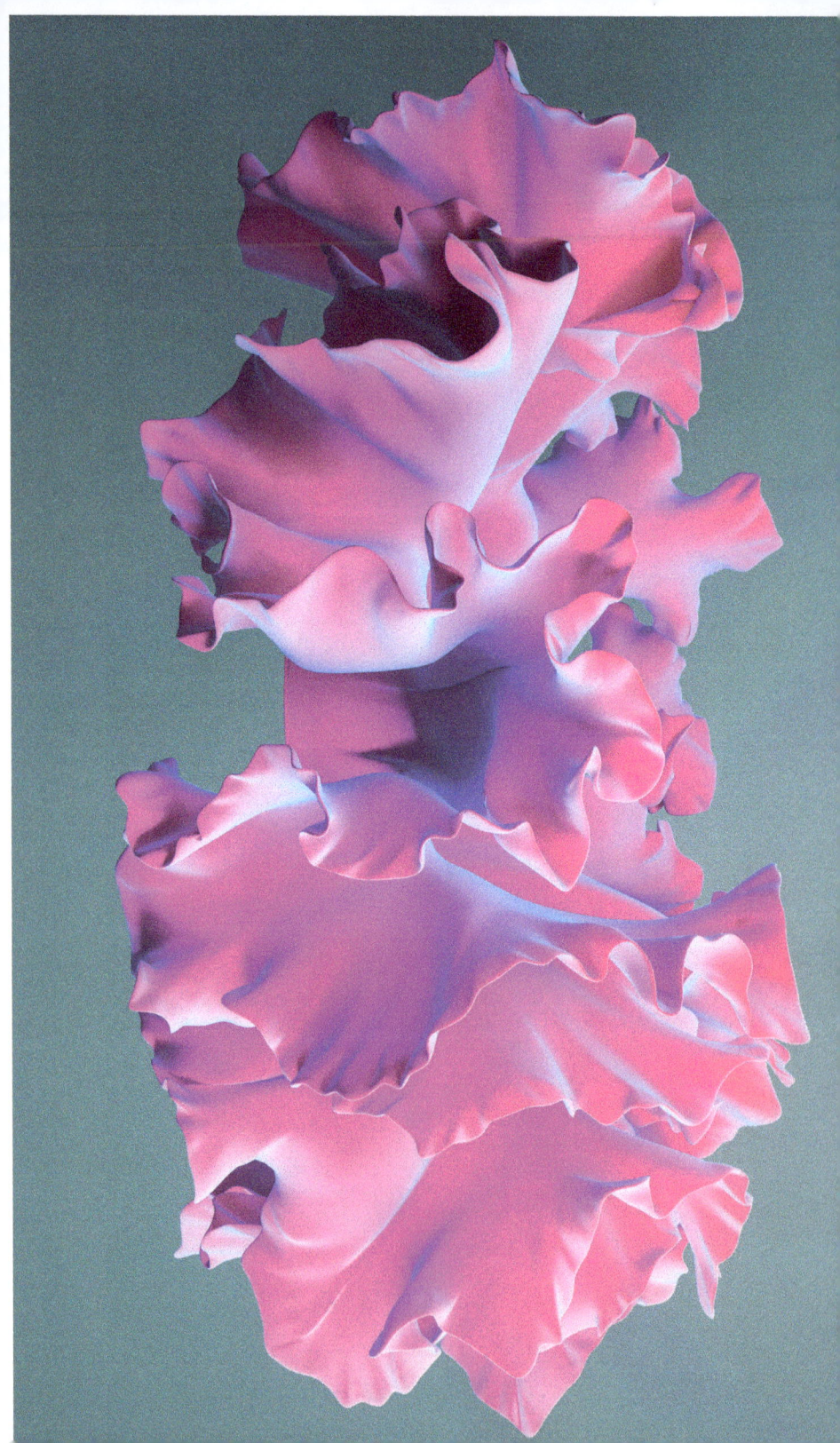

21- GETTING ALTERNATIVE STRESS RESPONSES ON THE MENU

Because most of the formation of our stress responses happened very early in life, and beneath the threshold of conscious awareness, most people are under the impression that they are set in stone. But this is not really true. Each of us possesses three distinct autonomic systems, and the necessary neurochemistry to run them. What this means is that although we may have habitually left behind a number of defensive stress responses, there is no fundamental organic reason that we could not learn to use them: most people simply do not know how to get them back on the menu. They are not *functionally* available, but this does not mean that the neural pathways undergirding them no longer exist.

It's nearly impossible to change something you don't know you're doing. And for most people, for most of their lives, autonomic habits of responding to stress will be like this. The responses are happening beneath the threshold of conscious awareness. The part of the body that's responding is just doing its thing. It's happening automatically and outside of our direct awareness.

So what has to happen for us to begin to become aware of these autonomic responses? What do we have to notice in order to realize that we are responding from our autonomic repertoire?

Catching an autonomic response is a little bit like trying to catch the wind in a net. At first, it's almost impossible to catch it directly. But in the same way that you can see the way that the wind is pushing through a net, even if you can't trap it, the trace left by an autonomic response is often more obvious. And we can learn to listen for these traces. Some of them are left in the mind, some of them are left in the body.

INTERNAL DIALOGUE

If we find, in the wake of an experience, that our internal dialogue has activated, particularly with an emotional tone, this is a pretty good mental indicator that something has happened to us autonomically. I sometimes notice that I've shifted into a fight response because I start dropping F-bombs in my internal talk. I'm not even saying this stuff out loud. But when I listen inwardly, I can hear that my inner dialogue is now punctuated with profanity. (Sometimes we are saying this stuff out loud, and then it can be even more apparent.)

If the background stream of our internal talk shifts tone, this is likely the response to a shift in our autonomic baseline.

CRAVINGS

Sometimes the trace is in the body, in the form of a physical craving. Anytime that we crave sugar, or fat, or salt. Anytime that we crave a cigarette, or alcohol, or sex. I'm talking about a physical craving that arises seemingly spontaneously. Like out of nowhere.

Sudden cravings are often indicators of a shift in autonomic baseline.

There is also deep intelligence in the *particular* cravings. This was something that was really brought home to me by Dr. Vincent Felitti. I heard him talk about this after having done a fair amount of mindfulness and therapeutic work with young men in juvenile detention settings. One of the young men that I worked with in my final role at a juvenile detention facility was 13 years old, and had been so seriously addicted to crystal methamphetamine that he had suffered a heart attack.

Crystal meth addiction is gnarly. People's teeth fall out. They have all kinds of extreme physical problems. Most of them end up with raging addictions, their lives completely out of control. At the time, I simply could not conceive of a scenario where doing crystal meth with those side effects was worth it. But then I heard Vincent Felitti explain that the first prescription antidepressant in the United States was in fact methamphetamine.

The young man I was working with did not have access to compassionate psychiatric care or a decent therapist. But what he selected from the street pharmacy was an expensive if costly solution to address his underlying problem. He had a devastatingly unstable home life. His caregivers were in and out of prison and suffering from mental illness. And he was suffering, logically, from profound depression. With crystal meth what he experienced instead was euphoria.

It's important that he didn't get addicted to heroine or cocaine or marijuana. None of those drugs was effective in meeting the deepest needs of his nervous system. What Feletti pointed out was that absent dosing precision, any pharmaceutical drug could become lethal. Double your dose of Digitalis for two weeks, a medication used to treat congestive heart failure, and you'd be dead. Self medicating with street drugs, my young client had a very hard time finding the dose that gave him sufficient relief, without keeping him awake for three or four days at a time. At just the right dose a medication can stabilize you: at twice the dose it can destroy your life.

Pay attention to the specific craving: that's what I'm saying. There is intelligence in what the body wants. Sugar, salt, and fat are required to keep the blood in the appropriate configuration for enduring stress response when adrenaline and cortisol are released. Get curious about your particular cravings, which have wisdom in them, and are likely autonomic.

MOOD

Mood changes are another telltale sign of autonomic shifts. If we shift on a dime from being at ease to feeling angry, or irritated, or agitated, or anxious, or sad, there's a fairly high probability that there is an autonomic shift underneath this.

ATTENTION

If the way that our attention is moving changes, this can be a sign of autonomic shifts.

Attention suddenly moving from being at-ease and diffuse to single-pointed can indicate a shift. Threat detection sharpens the shape of our attention. At ease, our attention is generally diffuse. Threat brings it to a single point as we search for the source of the threat.

Things suddenly starting to seem surreal can indicate a shift. The movement into shutdown states is accompanied by the release of endogenous opioids, which make things seem dreamlike when released in sufficient quantity. At first, this may present as us feeling just a bit spaced out. Forgetting where we put our keys: things like this. *Did I turn the oven off? Did I leave the iron plugged in? Did I lock the door?*

Since attention is downstream of autonomic state, changes to the texture, quality, and shape of our attention are often autonomic in origin.

Nearly all of the body's perceptual systems are downstream of our autonomic state, which means that if we notice perceptual shifts, a fair percentage of the time something has happened autonomically.

The general idea here is that there are telltale signs of us shifting into a different autonomic state, even if we are not able to feel this directly. Sometimes the signals are more severe, and more unpleasant. Two of the physiological signals of the shutdown response are inhibition on breath, and a drop in the metabolic rate of the body. If we find ourselves in a stressful situation, and suddenly feel like we're having trouble breathing, or we find that our heart rate suddenly slows dramatically, these are again both very clear physiological signals that our autonomic state has shifted.

Sudden indifference can signal an autonomic shift. If I'm doing something I care about, and suddenly just feel indifferently toward it: autonomic shift.

Autonomic awareness is necessary if we want to have any sort of agency in working with automatic responses. We cannot change something we don't notice. But as we begin to become more familiar with the specific defensive repertoire of our bodies, and the particular neurological signals that they've moved into defensive responses, we can begin to look more holistically at why this is happening. These responses tend to have relational catalysts. Whether the catalyst is a partner, someone in our family of origin, a boss, a colleague, an employee… much of what shifts us into defensive responses is related to the exchange of energy and information with other people. I would be remiss here in this category if I didn't point out that those other people can also be groups. *Men*, for example. *White people*, for example.

What Felitti's study failed to account for were instances of *collective* lack of safety. I'm speaking here about sexism, racism, homophobia, and other forms of oppression based on religion, geography, and class. Yet again, although these are sociological factors, they deal with categories of safety that are relational between groups of people. In this group, we could also place politics. When a political group comes into power and removes structural safety from particular groups, or from everyone for that matter, it pushes on the deep knobs and levers of the Autonomic Nervous System.

Any relational contact with an individual or group that impacts upon our embodied felt sense of safety touches the deep levers of the Autonomic Nervous System.

Something that I would like to remind people reading this book of, is the following: *you don't have to talk to that motherfucker.*[1]

I don't know who it is specifically in your life, but I know very few people with complex chronic illness who do not have at least one deeply problematic relationship, or relationship category. Sometimes the person responsible for the original wounding that led to the adaptive-at-the-time defensive responses that undergird chronic illness is long dead. But because of the way these things tend to replicate in time (epi-autonomics), it is pretty likely that you experience that dynamic with someone else.

Particularly in scenarios where the defensive response is one of placating, where a person has learned to turn toward, and be available to an Other who is trying to do them existential harm, the ability to set boundaries and terminate relationships is a crucial skill for people with complex chronic illness to learn. One of the things that is generally valuable, by which I mean valuable across the board, for people with complex chronic illness, is to learn an emphatic 'No'.

The 'No' can be confrontational (fight) or evasive (flight). Each of these is the arising of the ability to simply feel the energy of danger, and set a boundary. Either through confrontation (fight) or by leaving (flight).

---

1 Or those motherfuckers.

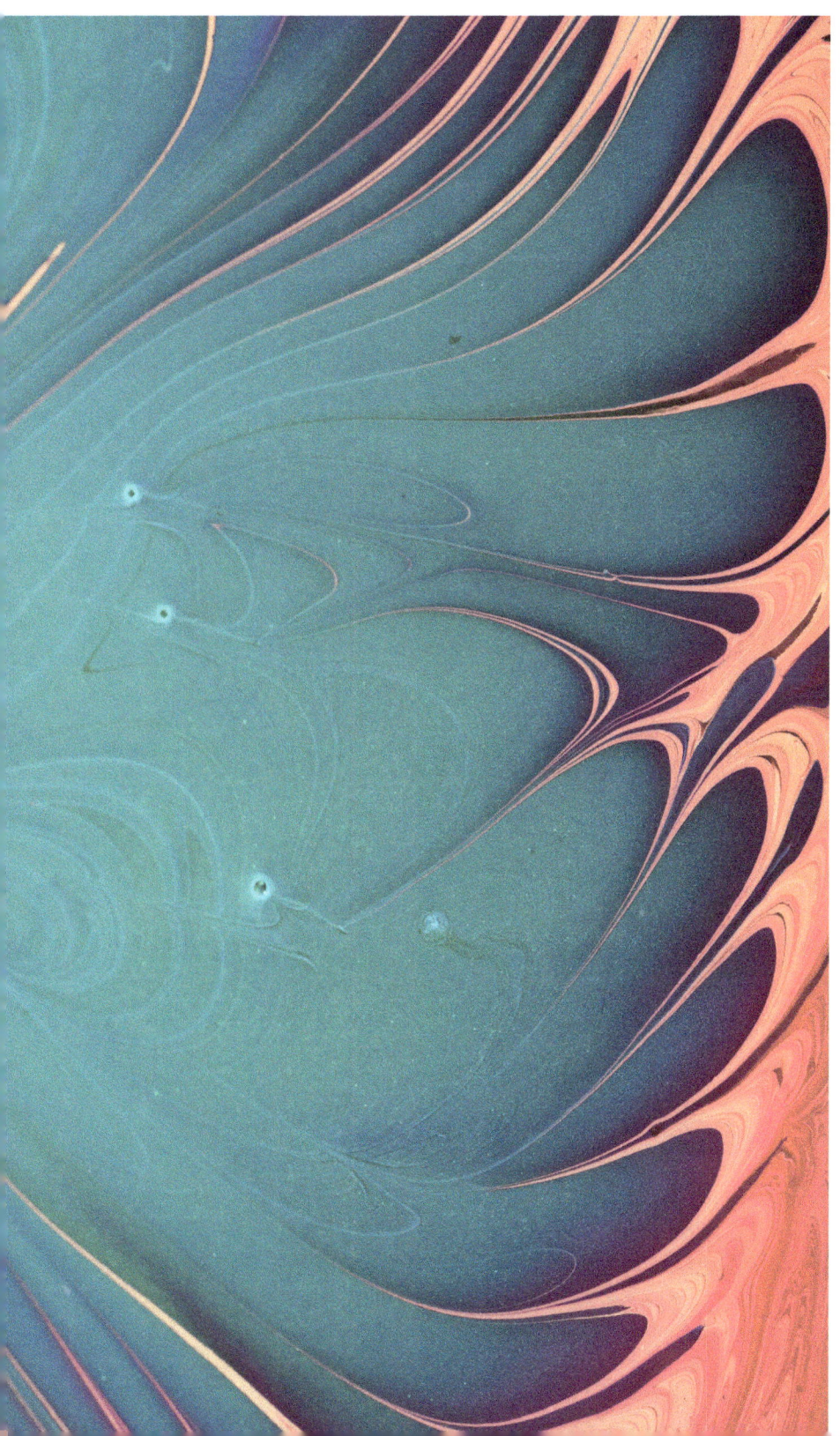

22- BOUNDARY SETTING AND CHRONIC ILLNESS

I was raised in a household where there was a high value placed on empathy. While empathy is a very important quality to cultivate, and while it's unquestionably necessary for us to be able to look at events and experiences from someone else's perspective, as much as possible, there are times when empathy is indicated, and times when it is not.

Empathy is not indicated when someone is trying to actively harm you. When someone is trying to actively harm you, boundaries are indicated. It does not matter why they are trying to harm you. It does not matter if you can understand how the difficulties they've been through, the things they have suffered, are causing them to try to harm you. I don't care about any of that, and neither should you. Because the thing I can pretty much guarantee you is that it is not easy for you to set a boundary.

And what I can also guarantee you is that the person who is trying to hurt you knows this, can feel it, and is exploiting that, whether they are doing so consciously or not. Empathy for people with personality disorders, narcissistic tendencies, sociopaths, psychopaths, people who are power-seeking, and seeking power over, is simply not a good idea. Those are the people that you should tell to get the fuck away from you.

Most of the people that I know with complex chronic illness have an extremely hard time setting firm boundaries. Most of them, when we drill into this, also have really elaborate intellectual justifications for not having clear boundaries.

Sometimes the justifications are religious or moral. They have to do with ideas about what it means to be a good person. *Well, Jesus never turned away from anyone.* Or they have to do with the person's sense of compassion. *There are two sides to every story.* Or their sense of loyalty. *Loyalty is the highest virtue.* Or with deeply held ideas about what family does, or does not do. *Blood is thicker than water.* Often these ideas are so deeply held, so core to the person's worldview, that they are simply enshrined in aphorism. They have become inwardly solidified; reside in a place that cannot be touched and is immune to examination. I would like to strongly suggest that you ask yourself where, and from whom, you learned these justifications. And I would like to ask you to carefully examine who they benefit.

The choice, as someone gets more and more sick, becomes increasingly stark. You can either learn to set a clear boundary, or you can die. To put it bluntly, if someone is serially violating your boundaries, they are feeding off of your life force. Often certain kinds of people do this totally unconsciously, but that doesn't make it any more OK.

People who have a hard time setting clear boundaries have a hard time experiencing their own disgust. I want to help you develop the capacity to experience disgust with the people who are feeding off of you. I don't want you to empathize with them. I don't want you to tell me a story about why they had it so hard as children, and therefore need to cannibalize your life force. Or that they are not doing it on purpose. Or that they cannot handle your rejection. Or that they don't really understand what love is. Or that they need you. Or that you are the only person who understands them. It doesn't matter why they are feeding off your life force. I just want them to stop. So should you.

If you woke up this morning, walked into a medical office, and went into a scanning device that showed you that you had a giant parasitic worm in your guts, would you feel empathy for the worm? Would you feel profoundly hesitant to kill it, or get it out of your body, knowing that you were depriving it of the nourishment it needed in order to survive? No, you would not. You would be completely disgusted, and you would do every-

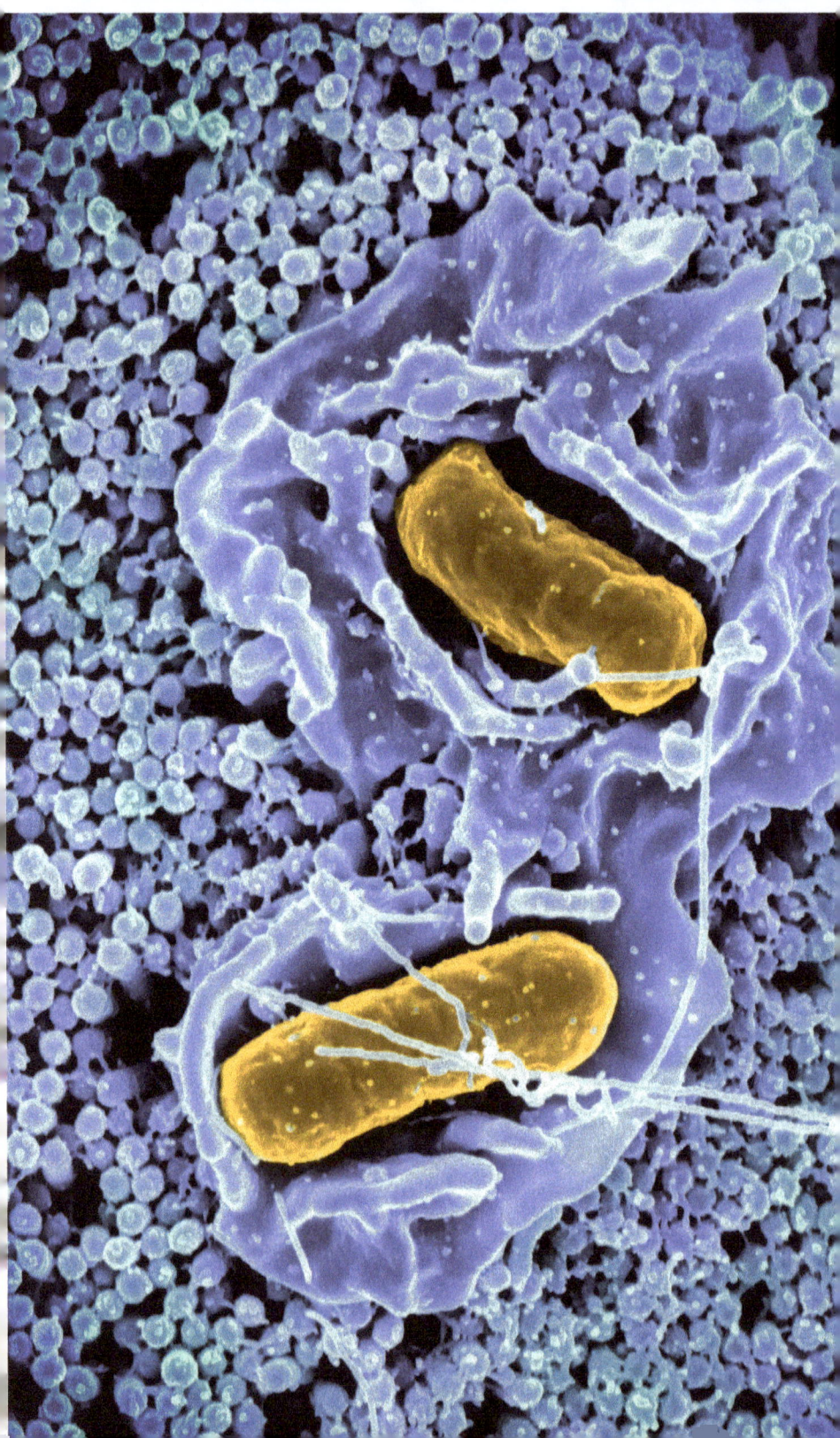

thing in your power to kill that thing and flush it out of your body as quickly as possible. I would like you to do the same thing with parasitic worms that are not inside your body.

Let us dwell upon this notion of parasitic worms for a moment, because as disgusting as the image is, the co-infections– Lyme, tick-born illness, mold, et cetera, are all forms of parasitism. These are all other organisms that have taken up residence within you to feed off your life force. What I would like you to consider, for a moment, is the amount of effort that you are currently making, in your healing journey, to eliminate parasites inside your body.

I would like you to consider why you are not making a parallel effort to eliminate parasites outside of your body? Who is feeding on your life force but does not reside within your body? And is it possible that your inability or unwillingness to stop this, your inability to erect a boundary that prevents people outside of you from feeding off of you is in fact the exact same process that is creating the opening for other organisms to feed off you from inside? Because here we begin to get at the crux of chronic illness.

Chronic illness happens when there is a mismatch between the degree and kind of threat, and our autonomic and immune responses to it. When we welcome lifethreats, and have lifethreat responses to things that are not dangerous.

Eighty percent of your immune system's cells are in your guts. One of the primary neurobiological sequelae of the shutdown response is in shutting down the guts. What is your immune system doing, anyway? What is it? *Your immune system is your biological identity verification system.* It is the biological system that differentiates between you and *not* you. Between self and Other. Between what is dangerous and what is not dangerous.

The purpose of learning to set boundaries with clarity is that if you cannot close the gates such that other entities are not invited to feed on your lifeforce, you cannot close the gates so that other entities are not invited to feed on your lifeforce.

If you denature your own bodily integrity by allowing other people to feed off of your lifeforce, essentially treating them as though they exist inside your boundary of self, your immune system cannot effectively maintain your bodily integrity.

As the energy processing templates of the Autonomic Nervous System go, so goes the immune system.

Do you understand what I am saying?

Chronic illness did not start inside your body. It started in the space between you and others, in the *relating*. It started, often, in our inability to set a boundary between us and someone dangerous to us.

23- NOT EATING OTHER PEOPLE'S WASTE ENERGY

In 2022, the firm that I direct began working with a functional medicine group in Massachusetts specifically focused on the treatment of Mast Cell Activation Syndrome (MCAS). Most of their patients had a history of a decade or more of chronic symptomology, and most of them shared in common profound challenges finding effective relief through allopathic medicine. Many had been on long and arduous medical journeys, shuffled through a system that dismissed their symptoms, marginalized them, and couldn't provide them pathways back to wellbeing.

We were working with their Director of Research to integrate our autonomics framework into their clinical treatment model: developing a curriculum sequence for their patients, and I was excited to have the opportunity to see how supporting autonomic awareness would accelerate their healing trajectories. I had trained their Director of Mindbody Therapies, and was excited to learn with them about supporting their patients.

Demographically, their patient population skewed heavily female. I didn't find this particularly surprising, because the autonomic configuration most typically underlying MCAS is *placating*. This variant of the appease response is something that women in our culture are taught to do more than men.[2] A lot of the messaging for women around what it means to be a good person involves preserving relationships and care-taking. What this often means is that women are statistically more likely than men to stay open towards others who are causing them harm.

---

2 It is something that groups who are less sociologically centered are taught to do more than groups that are more sociologically centered. This is a broader social issue that relates to the power dynamics of domination systems.

While affiliative responses can be healthy and adaptive in certain contexts[3], and encompass the range of responses known as tend-and-befriend, they also have more pathogenic formulations, particularly in more individualistic cultures.[4] Both the appease response, and placating, *if they become default defensive autonomic habits,* are linked to the development of various kinds of auto-immune dysfunction, migraines, and fibromyalgia. *Appease* is the use of sociality, and social engagement neurology, atop a fundamental neuroception of danger. You can think of it as a blend of sociality overlaid on top of a fight-or-flight response. Placating is a more extreme version of this, where sociality is overlaid on top of a shutdown response.

Both of these responses put the body into conflict with itself both neurologically and neurochemically. Since the role of social engagement is to connect, and the role of fight-or-flight is to set a boundary, you can see how trying to simultaneously open to somebody and set a boundary would cause a biological paradox. Furthermore, when we talk about placating, and the movement into a lifethreat response, the shutdown response is characterized in part by boundaries becoming increasingly permeable. So again, we have a situation where the body is placed into a biological paradox, where one of the impulses is to open while the other is to vacate. If you open and vacate simultaneously, there is space inside you for someone else to invade you (see the previous chapter on parasitic worms).

While I was not particularly surprised to learn that most of the clinic's patient population was female, the next thing I learned from the Director of Research astonished me. What she mentioned, somewhat casually, was that 50% of their patient

---

3 Parenting and care-giving both often involve long-term affiliative asymmetries. We are caring for people (either little ones, older ones, or sick ones) who are unable to reciprocate relationally, and whose behavior may at times be causing us harm, and yet to whom we need to stay connected.

4 See the work of Dr. Niloufer Merchant for interesting inquiries into the difference between appeasing in individualistic versus collectivist cultures.

population had a parent with a personality disorder.

This stopped me in my tracks. The clinic is not particularly large. But any time that 50% of a clinical population with a shared disease has a characteristic in common, it's really worth looking at what that might mean. Personality disorders are fundamentally disorders of relating. The DSM-V recognizes nine distinct categories of personality disorder. Although it comes in different flavors, each of these disorders distills down to the person having a fundamental inability to metabolize their own emotions.

The relationship between Mast Cell Activation Syndrome, and having a parent with a personality disorder becomes perfectly obvious once we understand this. If a parent has emotions that they cannot metabolize, where do they put them? The answer often is that they install them in the child.

I've heard a joke made, the substance of which asks the following question: *Why are your parents able to so easily push your buttons?* The answer: *They were the ones who installed them.*

The joke is a little bit flippant, but the point it's making is quite serious. We learn autonomic habits from our parents. We learn what it means to be who we are through relational contact: through processes of merging and differentiating. If one of our primary caregivers has a personality disorder, and cannot metabolize their own emotions, the emotions are essentially residing *around* them. Children, who are porous by definition, who do not have the capacity in the earliest developmental stages to solidify a boundary, often become the unwitting receptacles of this unmetabolized parental emotional content.

At a certain point in their developmental trajectory, often sensitive children realize that they can use their own bodies as a sort of storage medium for toxic emotions in the family. I don't think any child ever really does this by choice. I think the calculus is more primal and survival-based. If we are dependent on unpredictable and unstable caregivers, yet aware that we cannot survive without them, we learn pretty quickly to take their emotional temperature, and to engage with them in ways that help to stabilize them. You can see very quickly how this dynamic, established early in life, directs a child who is experiencing relational danger to put their attention on the caregiver who is outside of them, rather than on their own internal landscape of danger responses. Rather than the simplicity of turning to a fight-or-flight response that would set a boundary through confrontation or evasion, a child dependent on an unstable parent must stay in proximity to the parent. Fighting and fleeing are not viable strategies.

Children in these cases learn to absorb toxic parental energies, learn to self-sedate in order to endure the presence of toxic parents, not through some cognitive process, not because they're thinking about it, but simply out of survival necessity. The extraordinarily high correlation between this early life experience, and the development of a very specific class of auto-immune disorder is surely not accidental or anecdotal.

If the milk you were fed as an infant had a certain quantity of poison in it, and you could not survive without the milk, you would drink poisoned milk. This is one way of understanding what happens to these children. If you develop the autonomic expectation that milk with a little bit of poison in it is the way that milk is supposed to taste, when you drink milk without poison in it, the milk tastes funny.

What I would hypothesize here, but have no proof of, is that a statistically large percentage of the parents of these patients with Mast Cell Activation Syndrome, who had personality disorders, in turn themselves had parents with personality disorders. I think what we are seeing here is the epi-autonomic multi-generational transmission of trauma.

This has been called different things at different points in history, with clusters of diffuse immunological, endocrine, and neurological symptoms aggregating together, and making their way through family trees. These maladies have always existed. They have always included both physical and psychological components, have always proved elusive to mainstream medicine, have been difficult to treat, and have always lived close to home. They are disorders that can sometimes be veiled in polite company, are not obvious in public-facing roles, but hew closer to home and hearth and disproportionately impact the people most proximate.

If you are an angry asshole out in the world, people just tend to give you a bit more space. If you are an angry asshole in the confines of your own home, the impacts on people living with you are more direct. If you cannot metabolize these energies yourself, often they are foisted onto those closest to you.

Many suffering the impacts of these illnesses, downstream of the traumatized and traumatizing, have been gaslit, marginalized, institutionalized, and sent to sanatoriums. The evil of white bodies has been bourn by black bodies. The evil of men has been carried by women. It is a great stain on the dignity of the human lineage that harms perpetuated by individuals and groups are born by their victims; that the oppressed carry the marks of the oppressor *when the illness is of the oppressor*. What an un-ending tragedy.

It is for this reason that I do not want you to collude with those harming you. Instead, I want you to learn to hold them accountable, both for your healing and for theirs. It is actually a great gift to the perpetrator to hold them accountable.

24- PLACATE

We placate when the body moves into terror, but it is still necessary for us to turn socially toward the source of the threat. Something in us has stilled, gone to ice, vacated, gone away, retreated. But we are still forced to be in proximity, to turn toward, to tolerate. There are a litany of relational dynamics where this autonomic response might surface.

As a small child, having to maintain contact with a violent or unpredictable or demanding caregiver, when our inward sense is the desire to withdraw and recoil. Having to perform sociality in the presense of someone who makes us deeply uncomfortable, or vulnerable. "Go give your molesting uncle Ted a hug!" Of course, no one says the molesting part out loud, but if the bodily knowing is there, and we are still forced to turn toward the person, placating is the autonomic strategy that allows us to turn down the dial on self, to vanish enough from the contact to be able to comply with this request. Even the more innocent-seeming, "Come sit next to me on the couch," coming from an adult around whom we do not want to sit because we do not feel safe or seen can cause us to turn down the dial on our inward knowing; to override our innate inclinations if we are forced to comply.

Manners– the outward presentation of decorum despite whatever contradictory things are happening inwardly– can reinforce this habit of placating. Of learning to turn down the volume on our inward authentic experience in order to be 'well-behaved'. The British notion of the stiff upper lip; the poker face, the accoutrements of etiquette in high society are often masking functions that acculturate us to override what we are feeling in order to maintain social decorum.

At an autonomic level, vitality resides with authenticity: alignment between inward feeling and its outward expression. When someone says, "Go give your molesting uncle Ted a hug," and you stick out your tongue and run for the hills, you are honoring the bodily knowing. Autonomically, this is a fantastic strategy: sticking out your tongue is a motoric expression of a defiance, the child's *F*ck No*. And running for the hills is the successful expression of the flight response: a successful getaway. This response feels fantastic, aligned, vigorous, victorious!

Yet this also deeply embarrasses your parents, and so if you end up grounded for a week, or worse: tracked down out-of-doors, threatened with consequences, bodily escorted up to uncle Ted, and forced to give the hug as everyone looks on sternly, adding humiliation to the squeamish incident, your body might decide that authenticity of expression is not worth it. As children, we are constantly running this autonomic algorithm of expression and consequence. What is the available behavioral repertoire we can express to keep us safe? What works in the family and context that we find ourselves in? What works at school? What works in the society at large? Some responses, valid and authentic though they may be, land us in much deeper consequence and so they come off the menu. If the survival response more deeply endangers our survival, we don't do it.

Without realizing that we are learning to do this, we can therefore discover ways to self-anaesthetize: to put parts of ourselves to sleep, to dial down the volume on our presence so that we can tolerate these exposures to things that, were we fully present, would cause us to rebel. To fight, flee, or shutdown. Children learn, without realizing that they are doing it, to modulate their own neurochemistry in fascinating ways. We can do this through the breath. We can learn to self-hypnotize. Can do it by holding stone still. This self-anaesthesia is chemical, make no mistake. You can learn to cause your own endogenous opioids to release: learn to make yourself dopey and disconnected. Most of us don't think about something like this as a learning process, and most of us don't realize necessarily that we are performing chemical self-modulation, but undoubtedly we are.

As children we have the distinct disadvantage, in terms of having the autonomy to follow our authenticity, of being much smaller than the primary decision-makers in our lives. For at least our first thirteen years or so, the people with authority over us (parents, caregivers) are also distinctly larger animals than we are, and so can fairly easily force compliance. Since this is the case, we, as the children, may discover inadvertently that when we are forced to do something that we don't want to do, something that makes us deeply uncomfortable, it is easier to turn down the dial on self– to just dissociate a bit and go away– than to resist doing the thing. And in this way we are creating a self-reinforcing pattern of learning to placate. Everyone has seen, or experienced what it means to be physically present, yet emotionally, or pyschologically, or spiritually absent. All around us are examples of people going through the motions, dragging a body around without really being there in it. Some essential element of self has vacated, yet the person (or their shell) goes on.

One of the patterns that I have noticed in our clinical work around placating is that authoritarian environments of all kinds tend to require the development of placating as a survival strategy. Children who grow up in evangelical or fundamentalist households. Children who grow up with strict disciplinarians. Children who grow up in authoritarian regimes. Where there is someone with whimsical and absolute authority who can say – *Off with their heads!* – in order to survive we have to learn the autonomic calculus of ingratiating ourselves when the innate bodily response is to recoil in terror or disgust.

While the nature of this authoritarianism can clearly be political, it can also be familial, or tribal. Familial authoritarianism in a patriarchy is often manifest in the absolute authority of the father. When one person has bodily authority over the autonomy of the others, the others learn to placate because simply shutting down, going inward, disappearing fully is likely to get you more seriously harmed.

It is germane here to point out that placating is an autonomic response that is in direct dyadic relationship to oppression. If someone is placating, someone else is perpetrating. To fail to understand this as a relational dynamic releases from accountability the violence of the person or party that is requiring the person being victimized to placate.

This oppression/placation dynamic is a foundational autonomic template undergirding enslavement, to which the civil rights movement was the broad cultural response. It is the foundational template undergirding patriarchy, to which the women's rights movement was the broad cultural response. I would be remiss if I didn't point out that the current political regime in the United States, circa 2025, with its clear authoritarian inclinations, is creating a context of systemic deprivation of safety that is broadly culturally eliciting placating responses.

Children raised in environments of absolute authority– be they the absolute authority of the father, of the state, or of religion are more likely to develop placating strategies as a core feature of their defensive autonomic repertoire. They are also more likely to develop an existential fear of annihilation, because what placating teaches us is to learn to self-extinguish.

I would like to end this chapter by pointing out that placating never works in the end. It is a brilliant and sadly necessary strategy at times, but oppression does not end because it is successfully placated. The Emperor was never placated into humility and goodness. Chronicity of placating leads directly to complex chronic illness in various forms. It turns the cost of being downstream of oppression back into the body of the oppressed.

We must learn to decouple the innate survival response (fight, flight, or shutdown) from the turn toward sociality.

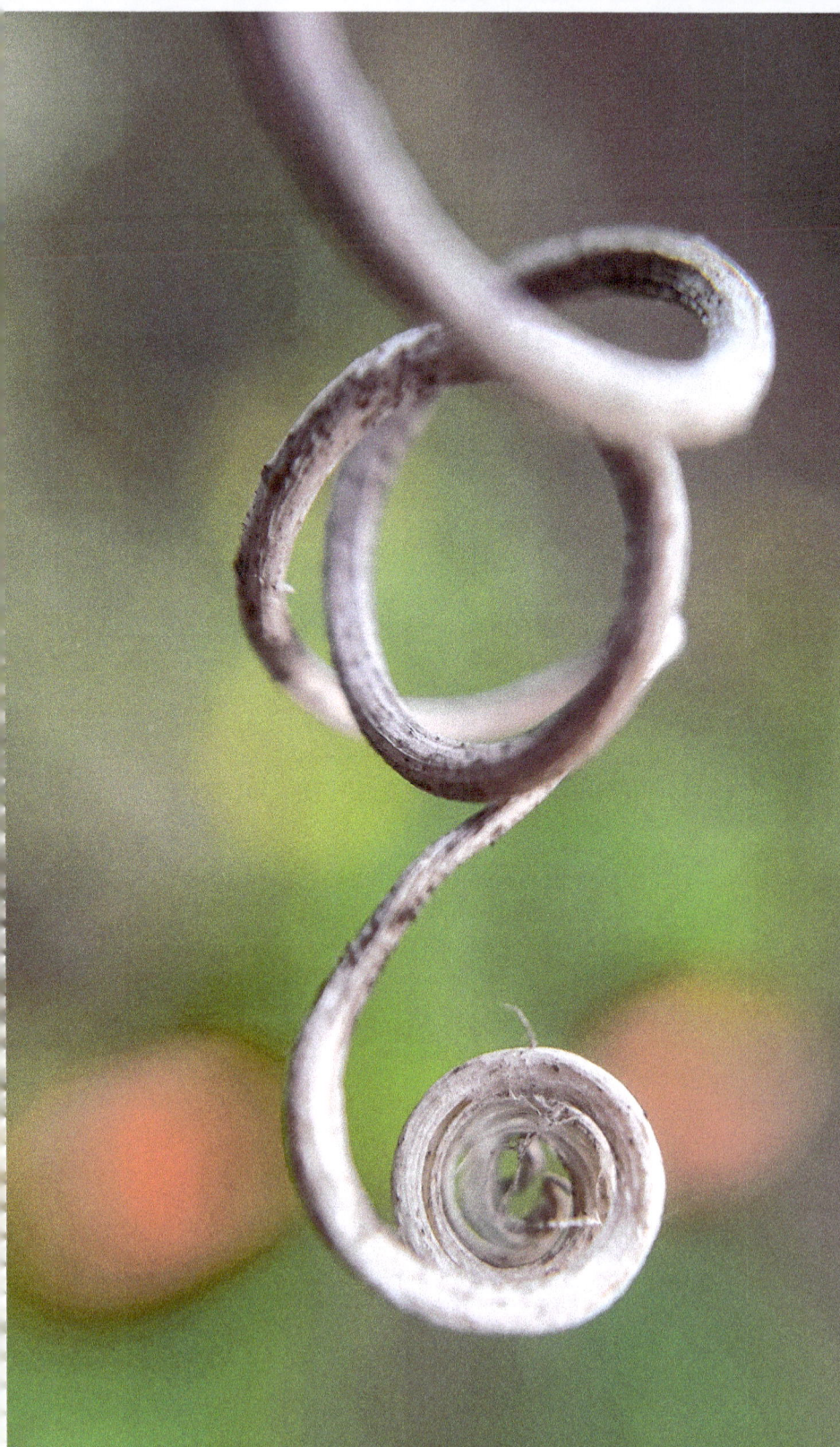

25- GETTING OTHER DEFENSIVE RESPONSES BACK ON THE MENU

In order to set a boundary, we have to have access to the fight-or-flight response. And for many people with chronic illness, when they listen in for the impulse to fight or flee, it is simply not there. So how do we reclaim this autonomic territory?

I grew up in a family where I learned pretty young that the fight response made things worse for me, and so over time it came off my internal menu of responses. The unspoken (and patently obvious) rule in our house was that you could be angry with mom, but you could not be angry with dad. She could handle other people's anger without blowing up: he could not. Losing access to my fight response was not something that I did on purpose; wasn't something that my ordinary sense of self was responsible for. It happened at a deeper, more subtle, more autonomic level.

As an adult, in my thirties, I studied Somatic Experiencing®, the naturalistic approach to the healing of trauma developed by Dr. Peter Levine. The curriculum section on the fight response was fascinating. Our instructor, Steven Hoskinson, taught in a way that was remarkably experiential. Several days into the training on the fight response, I started to notice that everyone was pissed off. Groups of normally studious and agreeable trainees had neared the point of rebellion. Everyone was filled with complaint about Steve. He sat at the front of the room, smiling as he lectured, the round dome of his bald head refracting the fluorescent lights from the ceiling, and yet as he talked, something in what he said seemed a provocation to all of us. Revolt was in the air, palpable.

I remember realizing, all of a sudden, that he was creating a safe enough space for us to get in touch with our fight responses, and all of us were directing them at him. Steve sat there, smiling, standing in for all of our dads, yet unlike them allowing us to point our anger at him.

When I was putting all of this together I had studied meditation for many years without realizing I was using it for state regulation, self-hypnotically, to re-purpose energy I couldn't metabolize. Allowing myself to actually feel angry was terrifying to me. I was a meditator, a calm dude, a peaceful guy. This identity prop conveniently allowed me to not have to address the core of the physiological dysregulation I was carrying.

One day, shortly after the training with Steve, I was driving on a windy two-lane road near my house when a dump truck came up behind me. The speed limit was 35, and I was doing the limit. The road was filled with switchbacks. I increased my speed a bit— now I was close to 40—and the driver behind pressed forward. Had I hit the breaks he would have slammed into the back of my car. There was so little space between us that I couldn't pull off the road, and I couldn't believe how aggressively he was driving. In the rearview I couldn't see the driver, only the front bumper and grille of the truck looming monstrously over me.

I felt something building in me, a heat, an expansion, as this happened. At a biological level, the fight response is all about being able to successfully defend our space. Here was a biological encroachment, and there was literally nothing I could do to make it go away. I couldn't pull off the road, which had a sheer drop on the far side, and no shoulder on my side, without putting myself in serious danger. My heart began to pound. My hands got hot. He followed me like this for about three miles, winding through switchbacks, riding so close behind me I felt like a wild animal being hotly pursued.

I had to regulate my breathing so that I didn't pass out. The energy and heat built in me, stronger and stronger, fiercer and fiercer, until my entire body was shaking as I gripped the wheel. My arms and legs were pulsing. We went up and over a small mountain, winding down, him riding my tail the whole time, and I felt, deep within my throat, a scream beginning to materialize. At first it was vague, just an intimation of voice, but once we crested the ridge it began to solidify into a ball in my throat. It got clearer and stronger and more concrete, falling into rhythm with the pulse of my body, condensing hot. I was awake and shaking with anger, and clear. As we reached the valley, I braked quickly and the truck driver slammed on his brakes, stopping literally inches from the back of my Volkswagen Golf.

I threw open the car door, wheeled around—I can feel it now as I write this—felt the ground beneath me, met the driver's eyes, and in one coordinated movement roared at him, with all of my might, as I pushed my hands away from my body, **BACK THE FUCK OFF!**

What I think, in retrospect, was biologically important, was the way that he reacted. As I gestured and yelled, the man, sitting high up in the truck above me responded as if I'd physically shoved him across the room. His body recoiled and his head struck the back of the seat rest and bounced off. I pinned him with my eyes for a long moment, and in that intensity of assertion of power, felt, flowing back into me, the biological energy of the ability to set a boundary: to defend my space.

The truck driver apologized, he said whatever he had to say, I watched his mouth moving but I don't remember the words; I didn't hear them at all. It didn't matter, because what had been liberated in me had very little to do with him beyond the visceral response.

I got back in the car, and noted that he waited a good count of five before starting up again. For the rest of the drive, he stayed a couple of hundred feet behind me. I drove the rest of the way home, and although it was about noon, fell asleep for several hours. I was totally exhausted. When I woke up, I had a biological response back on my menu that I hadn't had since childhood. That experience, of reclaiming my fight response, was worth the three year tuition of the course by itself.[1]

I have since that occurrence fifteen years ago had a series of other experiences that were about reclaiming and re-writing the autonomic habits my body uses to respond to threat. For me, the primary autonomic response I had lost was the fight response, and so many of the reclamations have involved this reponse. What each of them shared was a situation arising where I had to push beyond my comfort zone, and over-ride a bodily sensing of danger, to assert myself.

I'm thinking about two situations in particular, one of which happened on the tennis court, and one of which involved a confrontation with a neighbor, and neither one of them were easy. The confrontation with the neighbor, who is an alcoholic and a bully, was the most intense. Prior to that event, I had never screamed in someone's face. After dealing with a series of egregious verbal aggressions from this person, I discovered that my body was simply done taking bullshit from him. I physically confronted him, got right in his face, and screamed at him at full volume for about five minutes. I really let him have it, unleashing a string of profanities so acid and fluent it seemed to have been stored up from every experience I had ever had of being bullied in my life.

I cursed him with the fluency of a drunken sailor, stone cold sober, standing in the middle of a dirt road at two o'clock in the afternoon, told him to get the fuck out of my way if he didn't want to get run over and then returned home. In the

---

1 I want to acknowledge here my privileged social location as a White man, in relationship to this story. Had I been a woman, had I been a Black man, or had I been a Black woman, the interaction with the truck driver might have gone very differently. There are reasons of safety why some groups don't express anger. What I want to assert here, without asserting that I know what it looks like, is the physiological need for all of us, in all social locations, to have these responses back on the menu for our wellbeing. This work of reclamation doesn't have to take place out in the world; it can happen in more structured and facilitated containers with trusted others, but it does need to happen.

immediate wake of the interaction I lost my balance entirely, had to lay down on the ground while my head spun (the actual physical vertigo was so intense I could not stay upright), and spent thirty minutes shaking uncontrollably, while absolutely convinced he was going to arrive in our driveway, walk down it, and shoot me dead on the spot.

What I want to emphasize about this interaction is that in its wake I was totally convinced he was going to come kill me. It didn't seem like a possibility, or even a probability, but an inevitability. Thirty minutes later, when my head had stopped spinning enough that I could pull myself up to sitting, I was properly astonished not to be dead. Everything in my body had told me I had crossed a fatal redline: so thoroughly had my body been convinced of this that I had completely lost my balance.

Like I said, I had never done anything like this to another human being before. It was not within my self-concept to do so. My neuroception of danger was so acute in the wake of having done this thing– it so foundationally violated what I had been taught was acceptable behavior– that I simply could not conceive of doing this and not then having a catastrophic consequence.

But after another few minutes passed, and it became obvious that no one was coming, I realized that my neuroception had just recalibrated. **What feels impossible to us to do, what feels like it is not an option, once done, becomes part of our repertoire.**

I have not, thankfully, had occassion to go off on anyone else since that interaction with the neighbor, but I have certainly, several times, told people to stand the fuck down, something I would not have been able to withstand physiologically before this. And possibly as significantly, my body has been able, since that event, to withstand the intensities of confrontation from what I can only properly call a different autonomic composition. I still don't enjoy that level of confrontation, but it does not put me into shutdown.

I would be remiss if I did not tell you the end of that story, which is that I came home, and I went to sleep and when I woke up the next morning I began to meditate, and I touched into the place in myself that the experience had awakened, and then I began throwing up. It was about five thirty in the morning, and just dawn, and I stood outside in our backyard throwing up with intensity. I heard our neighbor next door come out the backdoor on his way to work, and I couldn't stop barfing.

At some point I began to realize I was throwing up not just this interaction, but every time in my life I had been bullied. I was throwing up a number of interactions from highschool, with Andy Plax, and Nate Storch, and Greg Smith, and Joey Mitchell. I was throwing up all of the times I had been unable to defend myself because my beautiful and sovereign body had been so traumatized at age seven by being removed from the place where I belonged that it froze in situations where I detected extreme danger, and I grew immobilized. I stood out there for a long time that morning, vomiting up a lifetime accumulation of the poison in the milk.

The point here is not my specific story: it is about the process of reclaiming defensive options that we have lost. For you reading this, the reclamation might be of the fight response, or it might be of the flight response. It might involve learning to confront, and it might involve learning to let yourself get away. In either case, it will likely be about learning to give your body permission to move again.

Permission to respond, through movement, to threat.

I pause to admire the elegant simplicity of both of these danger responses, in their clarity. We need to have these options: to fight, and to flee. We need to help our bodies learn to confront and to get away.

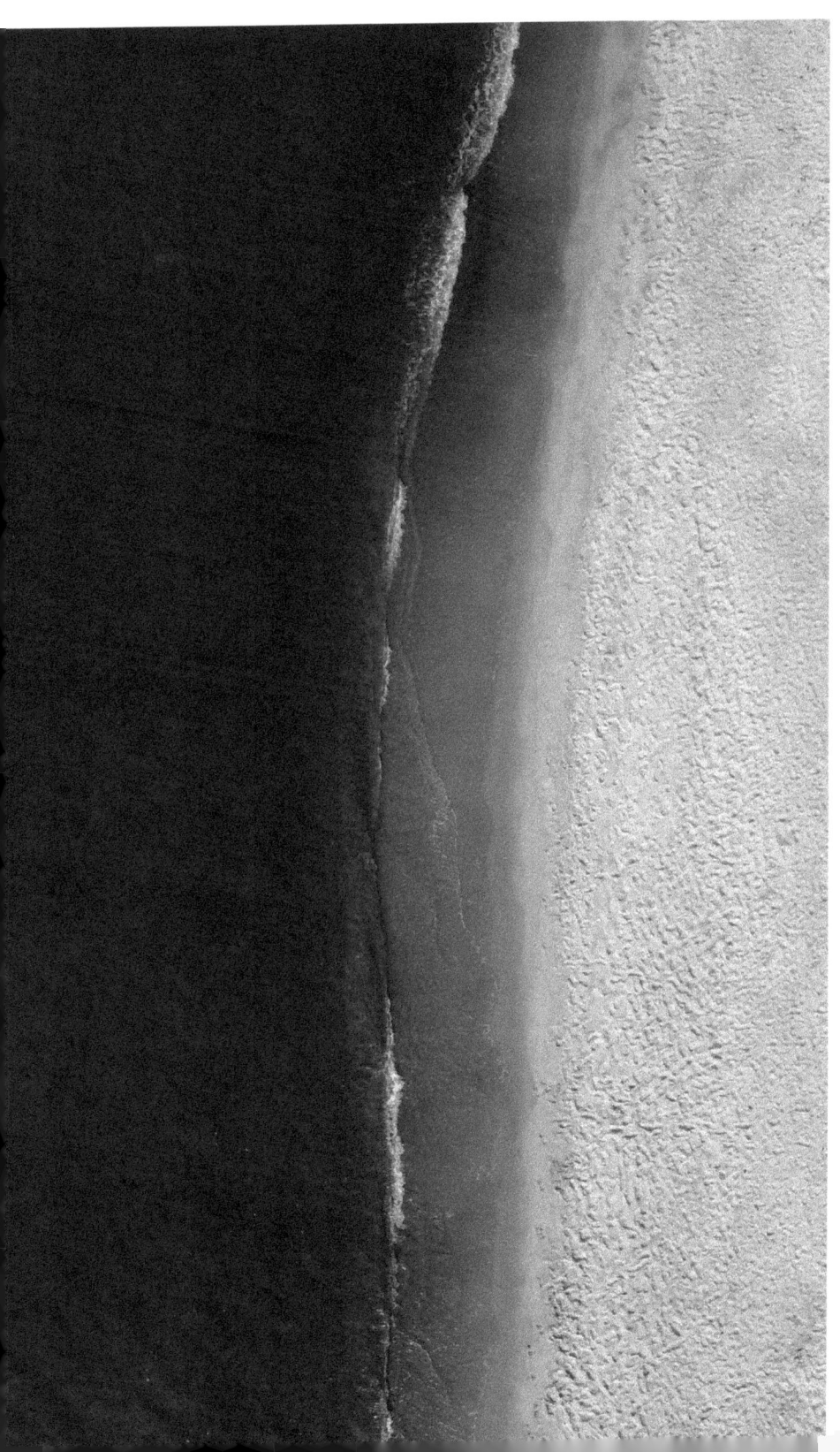

26- EVOKING CONECTION STATES

If we are dealing with the active symptoms of chronic illness, and we feel very uncomfortable in the body, it can be nearly impossible to focus on the evocation of connection states. Strong signals of discomfort from the body make it difficult for us to rest. So this third category of practice is not something that is very accessible when symptoms flare. When you're feeling better, however, or at least less worse, bringing your focus to the active cultivation of the experience of safety and connection is a way to strengthen the foundations of well-being.

Most people in the modern world are almost entirely unaware of the relationship between their daily experiences of connection and their well-being. When I'm talking about connection, through the lens of autonomic physiology, what I'm talking about specifically is getting our autonomic Connection System online. The interesting thing about this is that the neurobiology of this system is designed in such a way that it can allow us to connect with pretty much anything. For a lot of people with chronic illness, relationships with other humans have been problematic. When they hear about connection, often they think this means learning to connect with other people. But to activate the Connection System does not require relating with humans.

We can experience connection in nature, with plants, or gardening. Through creative pursuits, like painting, or drawing, or sculpting, or ceramics. We can experience connection through movement practices like dance, or tai chi, or Chi Gong, or stretching. We can experience it by ourselves, or with another person, or in a group. We can experience it in the city or in the country. We can experience it quietly or at a concert. The thing to ask yourself is, *What activities bring you a sense of experiencing contact with yourself in a way that you enjoy?* Like the defensive autonomic states, there are a full range of health-creating states that utilize the Connection System. Some of these are on the

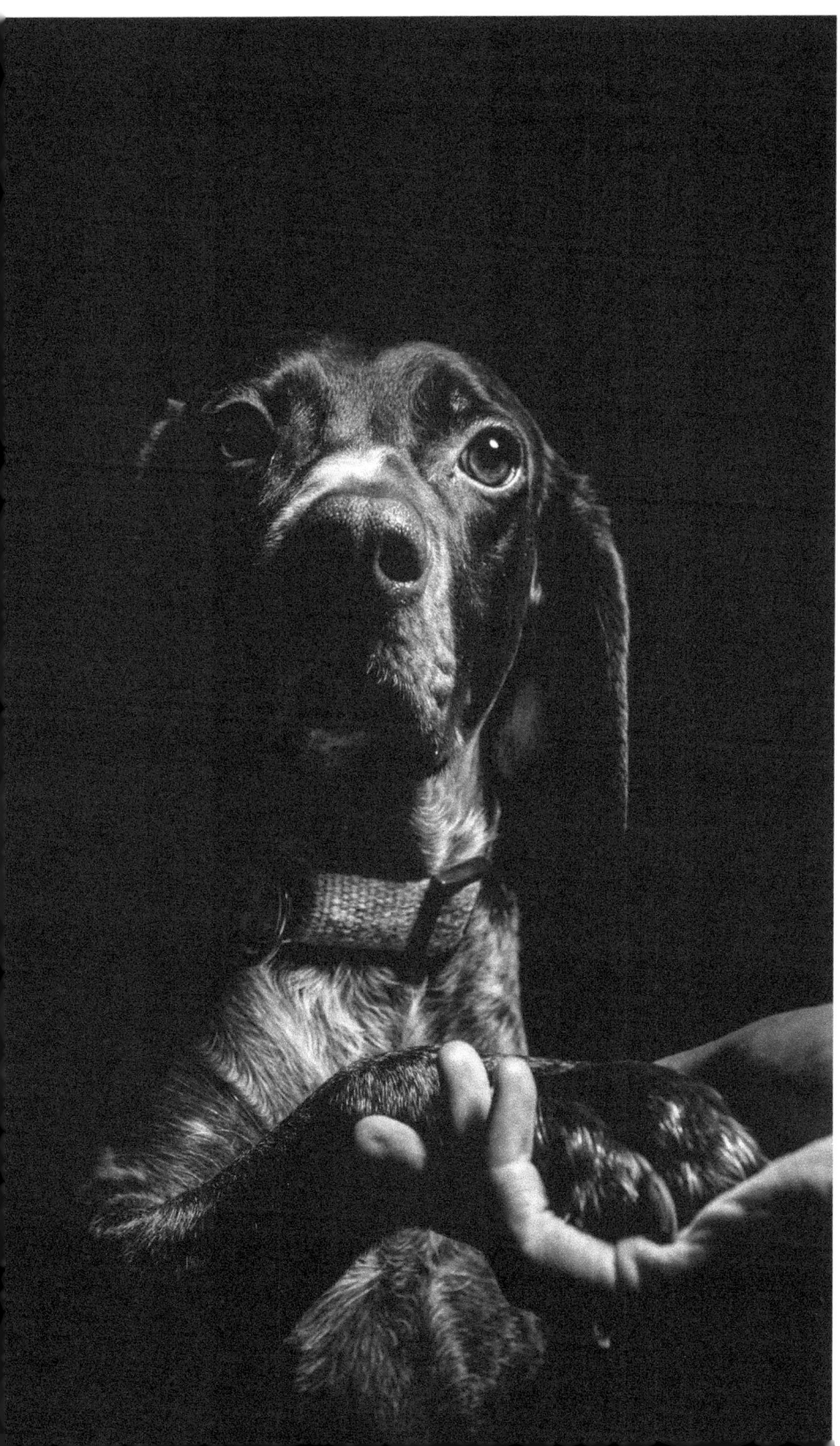

meditative side of the spectrum, some of them are more active, and some of them move into the realm of play and even competition. In the second appendix to this book, I've made a list of activities that is gathered from five thousand interviews we conducted between 2013 and 2018, essentially asking people what activities they engaged in to come home to themselves. I like to encourage people to think about connection as a form of food. One of the most important things that the COVID-19 pandemic brought home to me, was the awareness that most people do not realize the degree to which micro-moments of connection throughout their day are responsible for helping them maintain an experience of well-being. Unable to touch one another, required to stay six feet apart, wearing masks that obscure the lower half of our faces where most social engagement registers, we suddenly lost, as a human collective, all of these micro-moments of connection that are the ordinary texture of our daily lives. From smiling at a baby in line at the coffee shop, to giving your friend a high-five, all of the ordinary routes that we were accustomed to seeking out connection closed to nearly all of us.

About six months into the pandemic, I remember realizing that if I didn't find a way to nourish my sense of connection, I was gonna lose it. Over the course of the next couple of years, I re-directed much of the energy that I had been putting into friendships into connecting with the natural world. I'm not suggesting that one kind of connection is better than another. I'm just noticing that for myself, aware that I wasn't getting the connection nourishment I needed from my friends, because I couldn't be with them in the ways I used to be with them at regular gatherings, I had to find an alternative connection supply. During the pandemic, an enormous number of people bought pets. I think this was an expression of the same innate awareness that if we couldn't be with people, we needed to have some one or some thing to connect to.

27- CONCLUSION

In this brief volume I have attempted to provide an overview to help you think about and begin to approach the autonomic aspects of complex chronic illness, with the goal of gaining first a greater understanding of some of the deep physiological drivers of disease (the autonomic origins of chronic illness), and secondly a view towards understanding and transforming shutdown states (healing the autonomic components of chronic illness).

The book begins with the assertion that there is a dose-response relationship between categories of early relational trauma that shift us into specific defensive autonomic states, and the development of chronic illness. It observes that chronic illness, which we experience internally, in fact develops relationally between the patient (the person who is ill) and those with whom they are in relationship. It examines the origin of chronic illness in patterns of autonomic defense against threats outside of us, typically relational in nature. It reflects upon the way that these patterns of relating become habitual, and how if they become defaults, this can, over time, shift fundamental setpoints in our biology in ways that lead to chronic illness. It proposes that each chronic illness is actually an N of 1, arising at the subtle and complex intersection of autonomic physiology, the immune system, and the endocrine system.

It recommends the development of autonomic fluency: of discerning for yourself the principal defensive lifethreat states your body habitually moves into when responding to threat, with the assertion that chronic illness develops as a result of residing in sustained lifethreat responses of three types: *pure shutdown*, *tonic immobility*, and *placating*. It advocates for learning to bring back autonomic defensive responses that may have slipped off your menu of options in childhood: for developing response flexibility in the face of threats. It maps a pathway for more proactively addressing the autonomic components of chronic illness, within a realistic understanding of the way that this is simply one component of a larger set of systems.

My hope is that this handbook is both useful to you in building theoretical understanding, and that it is actionable enough to point you in the direction of gaining more autonomic fluency.

Clearly, it is really hard to make changes in our lives when we don't feel well. For this reason, I'd like to continue to encourage you to be really gentle with yourself as you are reflecting on the messages of this book, and how you might put its meanings into practice. It feels important to continue to notice that complex chronic illness typically develops over decades, and that the healing of it therefore takes time. The healing of it sometimes moves too slowly to notice, slowly enough in fact that it can seem like nothing is happening. And yet, even so, far beneath the surface, in the depths, the concepts in this book can help you to see more clearly the deepest and oldest patterns, often from early childhood, that have developed into distress and disease. Simply beginning to understand this begins to impact the patterns. At first, you don't necessarily need to *DO* anything with this information. Just let it settle into your awareness, noticing the places where you see yourself in the text.

It feels important to remember that as long as you are breathing, far more is right with you than is wrong. It seems important to remember that Nature is self-organizing and self-healing if given the appropriate supports. At this point in my career, I've had a front row seats to a great number of miraculous recoveries. People who have made their way out of the labyrinth, emerged from a dark night of the soul stronger, arrived on the farther shore. Chronic illness is, in a way, an individualized puzzle that each of us who faces it is required to solve. There is meaning in it. We can have trusted allies in the healing journey, but the journey is ultimately our own. The goal, eventually, is wellbeing– but the work of recovering wellbeing is learning how to find the wellspring of our vitality once more.

APPENDIX ONE: SOMATICALLY-ORIENTED TRAUMA HEALING LINEAGES AND INTERVENTIONS WITH OVERLAP TO AUTONOMICS

Autonomics, which is the living cartography of the Autonomic Nervous System that I have spent the past thirty years developing, emerged out of the intersection of a profound study of Polyvagal Theory with decades of immersion in awareness training and Indigenous Lifeways. It is an animist cartography of the Autonomic Nervous System, and expands our understanding of the *in vivo* functioning of the ANS, the foundational neurology of its systems, and the way that they combine and interact with relevant neurochemistries to produce the energy-processing templates that govern our moment-to-moment felt experience.

In addition to writing about Autonomics, Hearth Science, the firm I founded and direct, has developed an autonomics-informed diagnostic and treatment platform for self-healing called **The Autonomic Compass**. It is designed to help people identify present-moment autonomic state, and work (when necessary) to shift states in a more salugenic direction. On the platform we have an entire section dedicated to chronic illness. You can learn more here:

https://www.hearthscience.io/autonomic-compass

Because Stephen W. Porges, PhD was my primary mentor in neurophysiology for nearly a decade, and Autonomics developed to extend the functional cartography and interventions first articulated by Polyvagal Theory, most modalities that are polyvagally-informed have sufficient, if not nuanced overlap with Autonomics. We actually designed, and I wrote and art directed the Official Polyvagal Posters, which visually depict Polyvagal Theory and which I worked on with Steve's supervision for nearly a year.

Stephen Porges has himself developed two neuro-acoustic interventions that are licensed to the Canadian health technology firm Unyte. **The Safe and Sound Protocol**™ (SSP) was created to help shift the neurological setpoints of the ANS from fight-flight responses to sociality. **The Rest and Restore Protocol**™ (RRP) was developed to help shift the neurological setpoints of the ANS from shutdown responses to sociality. Both protocols need to be administered by certified practitioners: you can find a list of those at the link below.

https://integratedlistening.com/about/find-a-provider/

Peter Levine, PhD is the developer of **Somatic Experiencing**® (SE), a naturalistic approach to the resolution of trauma. SE is extremely effective in addressing the ANS components of shock trauma. Find an international practitioner directory below.

https://directory.traumahealing.org/

NARM, or the **Neuro-Affective Relational Model**™, is a somatically-informed mindfulness-based therapeutic framework that blends SE-style nervous system regulation with a psychotherapeutic framework to address developmental trauma. Find a practitioner directory below.

https://directory.narmtraining.com/

Hakomi is a gentle yet powerful experiential psychotherapy that uses mindfulness and somatic interventions to heal attachment wounds and developmental trauma. Find a practitioner directory below.

https://hakomiinstitute.com/find-a-practitioner/

There are numerous other body-centered psychotherapeutic

modalities that address the neurophsiology of trauma, including **Sensori-motor Psychotherapy** and others. There are adjunct modalities that are hybridizing with more autonomically-informed modalities, such as **Polyvagally-informed EMDR**. David Bercelli's **Tension & Trauma Release Exercises®** address allostatic load stored in the psoas muscles. Arielle Schwartz has developed **Polyvagally-informed yoga**. While I am not familiar enough with these modalities to specifically endorse them, they orient in worthwhile directions.

Look for modalities that are experiential, body-centered, autonomically-informed, and address developmental trauma.

If you are working with a somatically-oriented practitioner, it is important to do this work face-to-face if possible. Remote Zoom sessions are wonderful for many things: somatic work is not one of them.

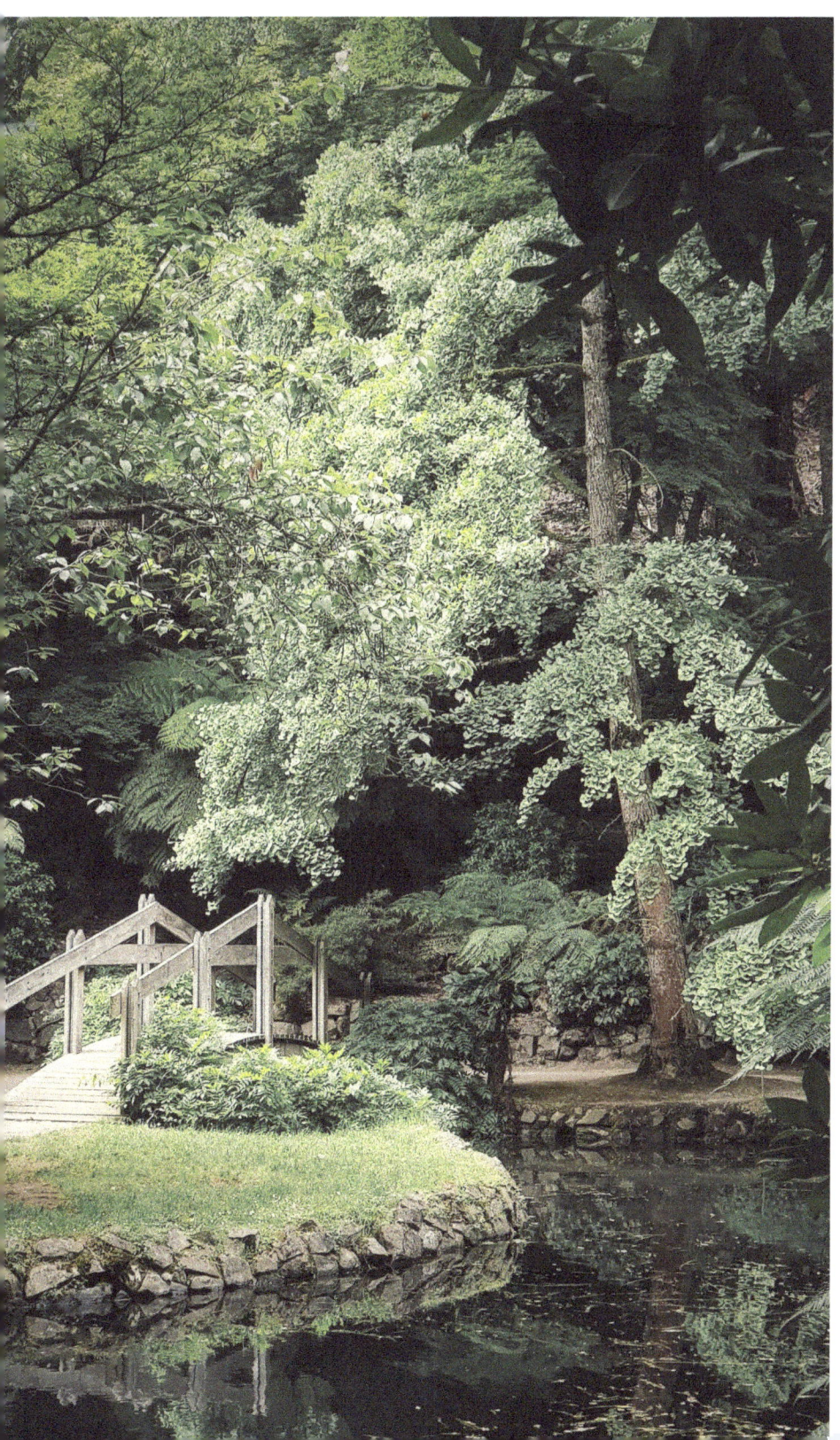

APPENDIX TWO: PRACTICES FOR EVOKING CONNECTION STATES IN NO PARTICULAR ORDER

Knit Something
Throw a Pot
Garden
Paint
Stare Vacantly into the Distance
Practice Gratitude
Stretch
Dance
Yoga
Smile when you Exercise
Bicycle
Cook for Yourself
Grow your own Herbs
Eat Seasonally
Forest Bathing
Learn to Breathe Deeply
Use a mindful coloring book
Play an Instrument
Sing
Savor Delicious Aromas
Ikebana - the Japanese art of flower arranging
Drink Tea
Visit a Farm
Learn Feng Shui
Read
Take a Nap
Light Candles
Stargaze
Turn off your phone
Buy a record player

excerpted from
Restorative Practices of Wellbeing

Take the Unpaved Road
Make a Fire
Open the Window
Forage
Balance Rocks
Do Nothing
Watch the Sunrise
Follow the Phases of the Moon
Learn to Prune Trees
Soften your Gaze
Study the Pattern Language of Nature
Mentor Someone
Burn Incense
Meditate
Rest your hand against a tree
Immerse yourself in water
Take a bath
Swim
Practice Quieting your Mind
Eat less sugar
Learn more about your ancestors
Learn more about the place you live
Learn bird language
Learn hard-ground tracking
Create an altar
Practice Gratitude
Surf
Use your Hands
Walk barefoot
Slow Down
Greet the Sunrise
Go Camping
Look up
Host a dinner party
Bicycle
Yoga
Look up

THE AUTONOMIC COMPASS

QUITE POSSIBLY
THE WORLD'S MOST SOPHISTICATED SELF-HEALING PLATFORM

- ASSESS AUTONOMIC LANDSCAPE WITH TAILORED DIAGNOSTICS
- TAILOR PRACTICES TO MEET NEEDS OF YOUR NERVOUS SYSTEM
- HUNDREDS OF PRACTICES, DOZENS OF EDUCATIONAL FILMS
- TEACHERS FROM AROUND THE WORLD

This work feels like a foundational piece of wellness and overall health that I feel has long been missing from the medical conversation. I love how it is based in the science of how we function- it is very practical, very direct. I've witnessed its effectiveness with my patients. These are places that I don't think traditional medicine or mental health has succeeded in reaching, and I find this work extremely inspiring and hopeful in its implications for healing.

-Nadine Burke Harris MD MPH, *Former First Surgeon General of California*

http://hearthscience.io/autonomic-compass

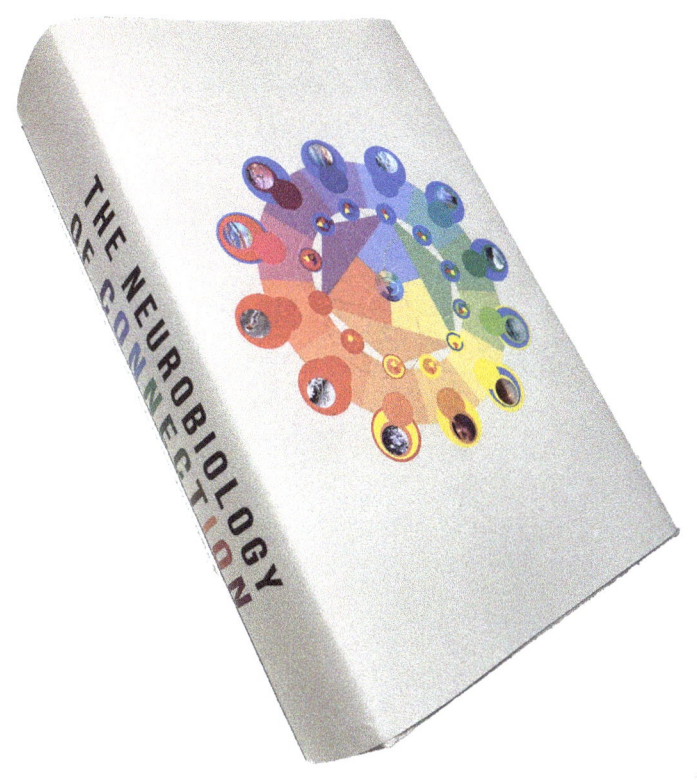

THE NEUROBIOLOGY OF CONNECTION
RE-WILDING YOUR DEEP NERVOUS SYSTEM FOR WELLBEING

In this tour-de-force from ancestral neuroscience pioneer Natureza Gabriel, the developer of Autonomics, learn to grasp and move the deepest and most powerful levers that govern your moment-to-moment experience of wellbeing.

Learn how safety turns on the neurobiology of connection, connection activates grounded interoception, interoception births intuition, intuition sparks relatedness, and relatedness activates enduring wellbeing.

http://hearthscience.io

ABOUT THE AUTHOR

Natureza Gabriel (aka Gabriel Kram) is the principal neural architect of *Autonomics*, a cutting-edge & ancestral update to our understanding of living autonomic physiology, which he has developed over 30 years of trans-disciplinary study and research with input from well over 5,000 wellness professionals, and 100 mentors and advisors from 25 lineages of healing in 24 cultures. His mind was trained at Yale and Stanford Universities, his heart has been educated in ceremonies and circles. He has spent 30 years studying connection through the lenses of neuroscience, mindful awareness, social justice, deep nature connection, non-cognitive ways of knowing, Indigenous Lifeways, and cultural linguistics.

He is Founder and CEO of Hearth Science: a translation research firm pioneering the union of neurophysiology and ancestral awareness to turn on the deepest drivers of human wellbeing. He is the principal architect of the Autonomic Compass, a proprietary diagnostics and treatment software platform that centralizes autonomic physiology in the diagnosis and treatment of stress-related disorders and the creation of enduring wellbing. He is Host and Executive Producer of *The Restorative Practices Film Series*, *The Connection Masterclass*, *Evoking Connection States*, and *Lectures on the New Foundation Model in Autonomics*. In autumn 2023 has was asked to lead the global Polyvagal Study Group on Facebook. He has been asked to teach Autonomics to people in 50 countries, executives in Fortune 500 companies, the faculty of medical schools, governments, international NGOs, and tribal leaders. He is the author of the *Connection Phenomenology Series*. This is his twelfth book.

He lives with his family on unceded Miwok territory (Bay Area) in South Salmon Nation (California) on western Turtle Island (United States). You can find more of his work, as well as that of the extraordinary faculty of Hearth Science at

HTTP://www.hearthscience.io

www.ingramcontent.com/pod-product-compliance
Lightning Source LLC
Chambersburg PA
CBHW052129030426
42337CB00028B/5092